You,
Therapy

RODGER DEEVERS

NEWMAN SPRINGS PUBLISHING
320 Broad Street
Red Bank, NJ 07701

First originally published by Newman Springs Publishing 2021

ISBN 978-1-63692-391-8 (Paperback)
ISBN 978-1-63692-392-5 (Digital)

Printed in the United States of America

The worst thing about demons is that they never stay in the holes in which you cram them. I don't know what level of understanding that you have about demons, but I've had a lot of experience and really need to talk about it, so I hope you'll bear with me. Now when I talk about demons, it's not in the traditional sense where an old priest and a young priest battle Viagrimelech the Dark Prince of Flacid, armed only with the Bible and their wits. No, the demons I speak of are far worse and much more personal. You see, these are my demons. I gave birth to them, I nurtured and fed them, then I bludgeoned them with some kind of heavy bludgeoning tool and buried them deep in my subconscious where they could do no harm or get in the way of my memorized mental recordings of 1985's Super Bowl Shuffle, performed by the Chicago Bears. I know, it's been like one minute, and I'm already losing you.

You see, I suffer from depression, I have for almost four decades, and I've recently suffered a setback, which is sufferer talk for I just lost my fucking shit. I had a total breakdown, and that is the reason we're here talking now because I need to work through this. I need to externalize my feelings and emotions, and I can't do it right now any other way, so I appreciate your understanding and acceptance. I know that I'm going to jump around like a meth fiend in a bouncy castle and that some things that I say will make absolutely no sense or sound like the incoherent ramblings of a concussed auctioneer, but I will bring it around in due course. I'm going to need you to hold all your questions until the end and silence your cell phone because we're fixing to get this awkward party started.

Everyone has a standard operating system that governs how they process and react to the stimulus received or mental cognitions outputted. Early in my life, as a newbie depressive, I adopted a system that allowed me to survive by "moving forward at all costs," push everything down, suppress the pain and torment, and make it to tomorrow. Keep in mind that when I adopted this system, I was thirteen and thought that Santa Claus was fucking my mother for sugar cookies and that the Bionic Man was a scientific reality, so I really wasn't really operating from a position of enlightenment. From that early time, my procedure in dealing with psychosis was set, tried and true—deal with it by bashing it over the head and bury it in a shallow grave in the wasteland of repressed memories. The faster I could move past the issue, the better. Tear the rearview mirror off; we won't need it. Some demons were harder to kill than others; they would keep coming back, and I would have to try and find deeper, darker places in my mind to hide them. Remember that time in the third grade when I split my corduroys from belt loop to butthole, trying to kick the tetherball like Jimmy "Superfly" Snuka, and everyone on the playground laughed hysterically? I remember it like it was yesterday, but I could never remember what happened the Tuesday before, so I would entomb that demon there and never look back.

The thing is that I was never dealing with my demons, my dark thoughts at all; I was hiding them, moving past them, hoping that the speed of life was fast enough to leave them behind. To be honest, I always felt this strange combination of both achievement and foreboding whenever I put a demon to rest or was able to wrangle my depression, kind of like when you send off your taxes; you're glad to be done but pretty sure not including one of the W-2s was a tactical mistake. So for decades, I've been haphazardly littering these depression-induced phantasmal corpses throughout my subconscious like an Oliver Stone movie. It was really only a matter of time before the hydration of a weary middle-aged man's tears reanimated long-dead grievances like Magic Sea Monkeys in a crappy aquarium. It may serve to point out at this particular juncture that my demons aren't "show up at night, take the batteries out of your remotes, and eat your babies" kind of demon, more of the episodes of dark mental anguish kind of thing.

So what happened? How did I come to lose my shit and find myself seeking comfort from a stranger? Well, it's never really one thing, is it? Like all my other losing of shit episodes, this one was a convergence of unfortunate events, chance, and like I talked about, the neglect of the past catching up with me. It happened just forty-eight hours ago. Forty-nine hours ago, I was the picture of mental health. I'm not really sure what that means, but that was me, just sitting there, looking not crazy. This year so far has been like the illegitimate love child of that time the Mayan calendar fucked the book of Revelations. It has been a challenge keeping it together, staying in business, quarantine, wearing masks, no concerts or sports, washing my hands! Then two things happened almost concurrently that would send me spiraling out of control: my son Joshua came over for a visit, and my bathroom sink started to leak.

A couple of important details that you need to know at this present junction: The first is that Josh is an amazing twenty-six-year-old man who happens to be six feet three, weighs three hundred pounds, and is severely autistic. Big J is nonverbal, and his life is extremely impacted by his neurologic disorder. His frustrations find their way to the closest human violently and explosively, often without any warning. I can't tell you how many beatings I've taken at his hands, but it's in the hundreds, with an *s*. Five years ago, J transitioned out of our home and into a house run by an independent living organization where he gets around-the-clock care and support, but if it's a Saturday, he's having a visit. I'll do a deeper dive into my main J Man later because it's a significant issue, but suffice it to say, whether it's consciously or subconsciously, if he's around, I'm on edge. The second germane fact to this theme is that I fucking hate plumbing. Let me rephrase that—I have a complicated relationship with plumbing. I enjoy and appreciate indoor running water and all the modern conveniences that it allows. I just can't plumb; it's like watching a penguin knit a sweater. I feel you looking at me that way, to answer your question before you ask it, yes, I know that there are people who work with and around plumbing for a living, but like most everything else in my life, it's complicated.

My emotional setback took place a few hours into Josh's stay. I had already made three separate trips to aisle 12 of the Home Depot and was awkwardly lying on my back under the bathroom basin, cursing like Andrew Dice Clay's parrot. I was an absolute wreck, running the percentages of getting caught if I just burned the goddamn house to the ground, when Joshua made this guttural grunting sound that I often heard from him before getting my ass pounded into submission. I'm not sure really what happened next. It was like that scene in *Saving Private Ryan* and every war movie since, where they are on the beach and time seems to slow down as your eyes and ears lose traction with reality simultaneously. My heart raced, I began to sweat profusely, my amygdala had fully hijacked my frontal cortex, and I was enveloped in anxiety. Not only did I think I was dying, I was hoping that I was, and that it would be quick and merciful, and that I wouldn't shit my pants.

My wife, Lisa, took one look at me and realized that something was more wrong than usual, and that's saying something. "What's wrong with you?" she asked. I couldn't answer, couldn't move. I wasn't even sure if I was breathing. Did I just piss myself? No, that was just bad plumbing.

Lisa stayed with me until I was able to respond with words instead of drool bubbles, and I was able to explain that it wasn't a stroke and don't call anyone, unless they bring an offset basin wrench. I gathered myself. My heartbeat slowed to a more human standard. My skin felt clammy but was no longer beaded with perspiration. I made my way to the living room couch, where I plopped down like a pile of laundry waiting to be folded. My youngest son, Noah, who also happens to be autistic, was concurrently playing a bowling game on his tablet and watching a show on Animal Planet and looked up with concern in his eyes. I motioned with a nod that he understood to mean "I'm fine," and went back to his business. I sat there listening to the importance of expressing anal glands, trying to figure out what new fresh hell I had just experienced and how to not only rationalize it personally but be able to explain it to Lisa.

Then the darkness happened. I found myself in a much more familiar but equally as uncomfortable circumstance; my depression had begun an all-out offensive. I guess there is something I need to tell you, and now seems convenient. I do not see my depression as some kind of condition, a chemical imbalance within the folds of my brain; I see it as a living, breathing maleficent organism that is trying to kill me. It is cunning and evil, senses weakness, and is right now laying waste to my defenses. I'm sure that there is a rational psychological explanation for how my depression manifests itself, but I have always had this adversarial "death match" thing playing out between my ears that nobody knows is happening.

Do you ever wonder why people who live with depressive disorders are notoriously "fine" when asked how they are doing? It's far easier to say "I'm fine" than "I feel an overwhelming sense of darkness and despair that permeates my being, my every thought. It is destructive in nature and threatens to devastate everything that I have built, my self-image, my personal well-being, everything. The evil infects my soul and produces hopelessness that can only be vanquished by the most desperate of measures. It loves to attack me when I'm at my weakest, and its sole purpose is to kill me with my own hands." Not only is saying "fine" easier; it avoids the clumsy moment after when the only question anyone wants to answer is "How do I get out of this fucking conversation without faking a heart attack?"

I have been dealing with depression for most of my life, and I have never felt such a strong upwelling of darkness; it was a storm surge that drowned out all other thoughts and emotions. It took a superior force of will to stem the tide, to calm myself and find some solid footing from which to mount my defense. I closed my eyes. On the outside, I looked like a dude on the couch avoiding pruning the hedge. On the inside, it was an all-out melee; there were circus monkeys riding unicycles, an old-timey steam calliope played "Aqualung" by Jethro Tull, while evil Teddy F-ing Ruxpin was burning all my files in oil drums. Anarchy ensues for as long as it can, hoping to find permanence in its effort, but even though the fury of this attack has taken by surprise, this is not my first hamster barbeque. I got up, put my AirPods in the wrong ears, every time, then put them in the right ears, went to our little sweaty workout room, and punched the heavy bag until gravity made the weight of the gloves feel like my hands were up the asses of small- to medium-size pigs, and I was trying to punch with them. I'm sure you get the idea.

Over the years, by not killing myself, I have built defenses that are more robust than many people's, requiring the depression to expel tremendous effort to not only take control but to hold it. I have accomplished this by establishing "circuit breakers" that will trip, forcing me to take more and more drastic actions. I know I piqued your interest there because usually when a circuit breaker trips, it shuts something down instead of requiring more action, and so you're wondering why I still call them circuit breakers, so I'll tell you: I don't know. Honestly, a good portion of my life has been just throwing shit together to get to tomorrow. Regardless, my circuit breakers are designed to alter my brainwaves from gamma to alpha; they are rules that I've developed to keep me proactive and managing my depression, that help keep me alive. Gamma brainwaves are the fastest brainwaves, not that these cause or are in any way complicit in depression, but it feels like with the constant, rapid-fire oscillations in feelings and emotions that they are a factor, whereas Alpha brainwaves are slower, bigger brainwaves present when you are calm but alert.

By slowing down my brainwaves, it calms me and allows me to regain an element of control. On normal depressive assaults, my outer defenses being attacked might merit the working of an art project or a puzzle, simple tasks that will adjust my mental course or attitude. If the depression persists, I will employ my go-to breaker, which is to put in my AirPods, crank some tunes, and take a walk, rain or shine, just walk it out. If it hits hard and breaches my citadel, I have to get a heavy sweat rolling and, like today, punch it out. This event, with the psychotic anxiety-driven mindfuck followed by all-out assault, is forcing me to do something I hoped I wouldn't have to do in this life. It tripped the mother of all circuit breakers. I have to get *therapy*.

When I said that word, you should have heard creepy, off-key violin music. It's been over a decade since I've had to "ride the feelings couch," but rules are rules, and some you only break at your absolute peril, so later today, I will be on the phone starting that process. I remember the last time. I had to tell the story to my primary doctor who wanted to put me on meds first, then when those didn't work, she made a referral to a psychologist who booked an appointment three weeks out. By the time I got in, I not only forgot what the original problem was, I was well on my way to creating my next set of problems that wouldn't bear fruit until I was out of care, being deemed "safe" for myself and society. Rules, however, are rules.

Do you know what just happened? I called the wellness center where my first-line provider works. "What are we seeing you for?" the friendly voice asked. I don't remember the exact word that triggered the response, but as soon as I said "depressed," "anxiety," "lugubrious," or "sad emo clown," I was referred to behavioral health, which was new. I called the number provided, and before I could say "I love the smell of Prozac in the morning," I had an appointment for *tomorrow*. Again, creepy violin music. It's a telemedicine COVID-19-induced Zoom appointment, but still, I'm not used to customer service in the mental health arena unless I'm threatening to harm myself, and I absolutely shouldn't be left alone with sharp things, or bread, because of the carbs.

So now I'm feeling some different feels. I feel accomplished because I was true to my rules and I did something I really didn't want to do, but at the same time, because of past experiences, I really want to blow the meeting off and go eat frozen yogurt with cut-up pieces of a peanut butter cup and actual peanut butter. Something profound happened on Saturday, something that has never happened before, something that, if I'm not careful, could be my end, so as my operating system demands, and if you're willing, let's move forward.

TUESDAY, JUNE 23, 2020

Good morning. I hope you slept better than I did last night. The suddenness of the appointment availability and the vacillating feelings and emotions that it caused led to a rather fitful sleep cycle. My fifty-minute therapy session begins at one thirty this afternoon, which is awesome because it gives me just over five hours to obsess about exposing myself to a stranger over the internet. I know that doesn't sound right, but I'm going to let it stand because it's edgy, and the caffeine hasn't kicked yet. I think back through a lifetime of dealing with this depression bullshit, wondering if there will ever come a day I can let my guard down, if depression will offer an AARP day or something, but I highly doubt it. I'm EFD (every fucking day). The nervous energy is building. Today I need a win because for the first time in a while, I'm scared. Saturday has shaken me to the core, has shown that I'm not untouchable, far from it, that I'm completely touchable. With each passing thought, I place more emphasis on a positive outcome of my appointment, which puts more pressure on me to not do something that I've always done—sabotage myself.

I have a bad habit of not trusting a process, especially if it's long and hard and requires constant sexual double entendres. I've always wanted six-pack abs, but tacos and peanut butter and peanut butter tacos. In reality, it's not that I don't trust a process; it's that I don't trust myself to follow a long process without shitting the bed and creating disappointment galore. When it comes to working on my personal demons, there is even more pressure on the outcome, which means the percentage chance of Rodger going ape shit, wearing a tartan skirt, and speaking in tongues goes up exponentially the longer the process lasts. To avoid this result, I will usually tell people what they want to hear, build a façade of understanding, then create a faux breakthrough, then walk out half-cured, still wholly broken.

Do you ever find it funny how fast time passes when you're getting a massage or racing a go-kart but how slow when you're undergoing physical torture, like having your fingernails ripped off. Everything seems to fall on that continuum somewhere. Waiting nervously on an important and stress-inducing meeting to start is toward the fingernail thing. My hands feel clammy as I look at the time and run through my head what I need to say, the work that I have to do while fighting back the urge to Google "how to become a mercenary for people who can't stand the sight of blood." I have been to a lot of therapists over the years, spending time trying to either please them or fool them, all the time having a running clock counting down in my head. The longer the interaction, the more I fear that I will screw shit up. I tell myself that every single first therapist meeting I have ever experienced is much more like a job interview than a therapy session, which oddly reassures me, even though I don't really like job interviews.

Not only do I feel this time pressure to "close out" personal interactions and processes before people figure out that I am a fraud, but my mind is also constantly trying to find a shortcut. I'm told that the best chess players in the world can see the game unfold many moves ahead, can envision their opponents' advances and counters, and can adjust their tactics to win the match. I don't know how to play chess myself. A friend tried to teach me the rules, but it just made me want to punch him in the face, but I did like the three moves ahead part because it illustrates the level of overthinking that I bring to any working relationship. No matter if it's a friend, client, process server, therapist, or sideshow carney, I'm constantly analyzing and strategizing, working the pursuit angles in my head to get from where we are to where we're going without disappointing the other party or having my head actually explode gray matter all over them. It gets exhausting, and I'm pretty sure it's either the cause or the result of a type of social anxiety disorder. One thing is for certain: it has made "living in the moment" practically impossible.

I sense your concern. Don't worry, it's different with you and me. You already know I'm borderline non compos mentis, so if I take my pants off and sing "The Magic of the Night" from *The Phantom of the Opera*, it would feel about right. I do have some genuine relationships that I'm able to maintain, but the number of people that I've let all the way in, that I can truly be myself around without reservation, I can count on my digits, and I have a couple to spare for a future snapping turtle misadventure. The problem is that the closer you allow someone to get to you, the deeper you care, the more you don't want to disappoint them. So when some cool, hip swinger cat enters your life, you're mind moves the pieces closer to you letting them down.

To be honest with you, I never really believed that by 2020 we would have flying cars or be able to visit pleasure bots at Le Martian Rouge. I never believed in the shiny cities of the future, even when I was a kid creating something harmonious and hopeful, felt not beyond human capability but beyond human ability. Now if you were to tell me that we'd be able to talk face to face with someone across town or around the world on small boxes with screens that made part of your face dissolve into the background while simultaneously making your voice sound like a droid passing a kidney stone, I would have thought, "That feels about right."

I decided to use Joshua's room for this meeting. Given its location at the end of the hall, it would offer a degree of privacy. I wasn't concerned about prying ears as much as yapping dogs. We have three large-mouthed, small-bodied dogs whose absolute delight in life is barking annoyingly at the worst possible moment. The door doesn't shut all the way due to being broken so many times over the years, but I propped it shut by moving a chair that's also broken, in front of it. I signed in early. Growing up in a house where five minutes early is right on time creates a habit that is hard to break. When you are in a Zoom waiting room by yourself with the video on its like checking the mirror, you can make sure your hairs on point, that your shirt is buttoned correctly, that your nostrils are free of debris and that you don't have any visible drug paraphernalia or dildos visible in the background. Now you just have four and a half minutes until meeting time, so you just keep looking at yourself, watching your eyes dart around. You can't stop, time has slowed to torture time, and you can practically hear the tick-tock of a clock you don't even own, all the while you can't stop looking at yourself. *For the love of God, make it stop!* Then, suddenly, you are not alone, and you're like, "Hi."

I immediately liked Dr. K. She struck me as a kind, smart woman in her late fifties who had an immense capacity for kindness and understanding but also wouldn't hesitate to call bullshit should the need arise. Regardless of rapport, the first couple of minutes are always awkward in the transition from pleasantries to business, and we were on the clock. The question was simple: "What brings you to my office today?" The answer was far from simple, and in the split second after she asked it, my mind was awhirl with scenarios and angles and overthinking and if I should just run away or tell her "Holy shit! It's a miracle, all of a sudden I'm cured, thanks anyway, hallelujah." After what felt like minutes, I decided to just start talking, just shut the fuck up, and start talking.

The challenge is context and backstory. You just can't have a superhero movie where there's action and fighting and explosions. No, you have to go through the feelings, what makes them want to wear spandex on a weekday, what shaped their desire to punch evil in the face, then the last fifteen minutes you get the action you paid the twenty bucks for. Having been dealing with depression since July 1981, having been institutionalized for suicidal thoughts and actions, raising two autistic children while trying to keep a family business afloat through turbulent times, two divorces, money problems, and a plantar wart on my right foot that won't die, I have some backstory.

When I had finally stopped talking, Dr. K looked at me like the chambermaid at the Heidi Fleiss residence. "Okay, deep breath." I wasn't sure if she was talking to herself or to me.

"First things first," she said. "It's obvious that you've been around the system for a while, so tell me what's new or what's changed significantly to precipitate our time together today."

I took a minute. I knew the answer immediately, but I knew that saying it would be difficult and lead to a challenging discussion. It finally just came out of my mouth, one word: "Josh."

When Joshua Grae Deevers was born, he was the poster child for poster children. He was happy, healthy, and a good pooper. He engaged and laughed and did baby stuff that made you talk in the slow singsong cadence that allows infants to completely understand everything you say to them. Around fourteen to sixteen months of age, we started to notice anomalies in his behavior. He began to withdraw from contact, attempts to engage him were often met with irritation, and his limited verbal attempts all but vanished, unless he was pissed, which seemed to be an increasing occurrence. By the time Josh hit eighteen to twenty months of age, there was no further doubt, somewhere the process had gone askew, and our once-thriving child had turned into mini Benito Mussolini. He was officially diagnosed at around twenty-four months, but by then a diagnosis of autism was a foregone conclusion.

We immediately enrolled Josh in all the programs that were open and available to him, read every article ever written and started him on a continuous drip of essential oils, threw out everything with gluten in it, and started the vitamin B_{12} and magnesium enemas—just kidding, about the enemas. Regardless, the challenges seemed to mount daily for J Man as the autism wreaked havoc on his senses and abilities. His capacity for terror increased dramatically as he grew. Josh would be calm and peaceful one moment, then transform instantaneously into a dark harbinger of death and property destruction. He would bite, scratch, hit, and kick, and over the years, he broke everything in the house, and I do mean everything—too many televisions to count, all our picture frames, two ovens, countless small electronics and appliances, doors, windows, my bank account, and my spirit on more than one occasion.

The only advantage that we had over Josh was our superior size, which quickly disappeared as he aged. The ability to understand each other was, and remains, by far the biggest hurdle to overcome as he has always been nonverbal. A man of no words, Joshua was hyper-resistant to every mode, method, or apparatus that we tried to open a line of communication. When he was in junior high, a behavior specialist with the school district told Lisa and me that Josh was the most severe case of autism in the county and that life was smacking him in the face at a hundred miles an hour. My son Joshua Deevers was not destined to lead an easy life; every step would be a challenge, and every victory would have to be earned because none would ever be given.

Josh bounced around from program to program. His lack of communication and violent tendencies wore out welcomes faster than a leper at a buffet. Life at home wasn't a picnic either for the big guy. He would be in his room watching a VHS tape for the ten-thousandth time, and then the tape would skip, or break, or just need to be rewound, and he would lose his shit and break shit and bite and hit shit. I was constantly walking on eggshells when he was home, trying to keep him happy, trying to limit the noise so as not to disturb him, trying to be "Johnny on the spot" with a snack or change of his tape. It was like living with a tiger, a murderous, nonfriendly tiger. As Josh grew older and bigger, the violence scaled up proportionately. By the time he was eighteen, he was six feet three and well over two hundred pounds. The severity of the attacks became much more intense, and it would take longer and longer for Josh to expend enough energy to trip his properly named circuit breaker and calm himself down. Josh once had an incredibly violent outburst followed by a grand mal seizure that ended with a trip to the emergency room. As the health professionals stabilized Josh by giving him a sedative, which took eight people holding him down, they looked at Lisa and me, both battered, an open flap of skin on my left forearm where he bit me, dried blood trails all over our bodies, wondering if they had sedated the right person.

I have stories that would make your sperm swim backward, if you possess sperm to swim, that is. Stories that involve strangers, police, officials from various state and local departments, firefighters, emergency room personnel, flying cats, holiday disasters, and Pop-Tarts. In 2015 we transitioned Josh to an independent living company where he receives around-the-clock care and support. Like I mentioned earlier, we bring him home weekly for a visit and to remain an active part of his life, and he hasn't had a Fukushima grade nuclear meltdown at our house in quite some time, which makes the timing of Saturday's episode so strange. I told Dr. K about the rapid heartbeat, the pasty skin, the sprinkler of sweat, and that I was clearly either dying or have contracted Vulcan pon farr and will have to fight a close friend to the death, which is really going to mess with my guilt issues.

Dr. K folded her hands across her lap, made eye contact with me across town, and said to me, "What you experienced is an episode of PTSD." This news was not wholly unexpected. She continued, "There is no time limit to PTSD, no statute of limitations on when it can affect you. Given the fact that you see him regularly and the added stress of business and life, it was only a matter of time until negative consequences manifested in unanticipated ways."

At this point, a faint buzz could be heard from somewhere on the dark wooden bookshelf behind Dr. K, five-minute warning. Typical superhero movie, just when it's getting juicy, the credits roll. Dr. K, not wanting to say "Yep, you have PTSD, see you in two weeks," but also having a schedule to keep, looked pained, noting the awkwardness of our conversation finale. In a soothing tone, she said, "PTSD is thoughts, your brain doesn't know that at the time, but it is thoughts, and thoughts, with effort, can be controlled." She told me that she would like me to do breathing exercises and start a meditation program. "Don't overthink it, just a phone app will do." I immediately appreciated because I was already wondering if I needed to find a "Swami" or climb a tall mountain and sit cross-legged for an extended period of time, because with my flexibility, that would be a deal breaker. After she assigned my "homework," we exchanged pleasant farewells, and just as quickly as she beamed in, I was alone.

I clicked off the program and tried to gather what thoughts I could grab as they swirled around the room like dogwood in the breeze on a warm spring day. A sense of accomplishment washed over me as I realized the significance of what had just happened. I talked openly and honestly about my life without elaboration or modification to suit my psychotic predilections. I found out what really happened this past Saturday, and I have a course of action to follow as a treatment. It feels like a start. It feels like progress. I know that if this was an Everest summit bid that I would still be in the town buying bacon and renting a mule, but it still feels good. I folded the laptop, moved the broken chair from the broken door, and made my way down the hall.

Lisa, my beautiful, supportive wife, who knows what was riding on this meeting, who knows my doubts, fears, and limitations, who has been with me through storms and fair weather, simply asked, "How'd it go?"

I told her, "It was good. I have a lot of processing to do. My mind is swimming in the deep end right now, but it was good."

She smiled. She knows that it's not as much what I say but the tone and spirit in which it's said, and you can't fake hope.

I gave up trying to bullshit her years ago. She's a battle-hardened veteran of depression herself, not living with it personally, but never discount what spouses and significant others go through in their support efforts. Sometimes I think it's easier to have depression than live with someone who has it. What Dr. K said about the PTSD and the possibility of control with effort clicked. If there is anything I have, it's effort. At the end of the day, I got my win, a victory that won't be celebrated in full until some magic time in the future, after I've put in some work and have paid the price to earn it. When that time comes, there won't be a band playing, a crowd cheering, or a big trophy to hoist up overhead while champagne rains down upon me. It'll just be me, smiling, getting to live another day.

WEDNESDAY, JUNE 24, 2020

I'm telling you, I went to bed last night with the chaff of the recently harvested memories swirling through my consciousness. Thoughts of Josh, my mom, who had passed away just a year before, damn pipes leaking, my first experiences with depression. I had a feeling that the ghosts of my space-time continuum would pay me a nocturnal visit, but sweet buttered monkeys, I wasn't prepared for what was to occur in the minutes prior to 1:38 a.m.

Do you ever wonder about dreams? Their meaning or purpose? Dreams have always been such a mystery to me. In the days prior to turning fifty, before I became legally obligated to pee at least once during the night, I would sleep seven or eight hours with nothing, hit the snooze, and sometime between 5:33 and 5:40 a.m., have a dream that spanned generations and felt as if it lasted longer than the movie *Lincoln*, which was a long f-ing time. I have had the "naked in class" dream; I ended up in a concrete drainage pipe waiting for darkness to fall, even though clearly I have nothing to be ashamed of. I know you rolled your eyes. It's okay. It won't be the last time, of that I guarantee. I have also had a dream where I was dreaming and woke up but was still dreaming; it was like getting sixteen hours of sleep that one night, and it was amazing. I know, I digress, and it won't be the last time, of that I money-back guarantee.

Let me tell you about this dream last night. You may have some insight as to its grand purpose or meaning, because I sure the hell don't. I was at the gym, but given my business attire, I wasn't there to get a pump on. People that I know and love are there, family and friends are there, but I'm confused because I know that they aren't members, and they're doing it all wrong. "Lift with your legs gramps, you're going to blow an O ring." Suddenly the lights go out save for a column of light shining down from above, illuminating a spot on the floor next to the hallway leading to the bathrooms and office. A weird tingle of foreboding crept down my spine like ice cream down a cone on a summer day as I waited for something to appear. Movement draws my attention away from the spotlight as the crowd of people begins to shuffle closer. I can no longer see their faces, but I feel them around me. The hair on my arms stands on edge as if electricity is building. I look back to the light and am startled to see a figure, a diminutive woman with Asian features locks eyes with me. Long, straight ink-black hair frame, her pleasant face, circular wire-frame spectacles rest lazily on the top of her button nose just above the nostrils, begging to be pushed back into place. Her hair disappears in to a black cable knit cardigan sweater opened to reveal a white button-up blouse and pleated knee-length skirt with a vague geometric pattern. She is not known to me. I have never met her on any side of consciousness.

I suddenly feel the crush of my friends and family pushing in from all around me except for an aisle directly between the unknown woman and myself. The mood turns sinister as I feel hands touching me, pressing on me. I feel confined and claustrophobic; air seems to be reluctant to enter my lungs. I want to run, but my legs are frozen in place. My wide eyes gaze back to the woman who suddenly moves toward me without moving her legs, as if she was levitating and gliding across the floor. Suddenly as she covers roughly half the distance, the light goes out, it's darker than a bowling ball finger hole on the bottom of the ocean, and I'm in the proper shit now. Excruciating moments pass, then without warning, she appears directly in front of me, her face illuminated from below as if she is holding a flashlight and screams my name. I sit upright as if my pillow exploded, my brow beaded with sweat, my heartbeat well within the aerobic zone. I know for a fact that someone stood next to my bed and shouted my name. I would openly swear to it in a court of law. I have never experienced a dream so real. What do you think it means? I know one thing for sure, if I'm walking down the street and see that woman, my plan is to defecate myself while concurrently running away. I may or may not be screaming like a middle-aged woman seeing Justin Bieber. I haven't made the call on that yet.

Needless to say, sleep was elusive the remainder of the night, not that I couldn't cross the threshold but because I didn't know if I wanted to. I'm sure I could make up a story in the morning for when Lisa asked me what I was doing holding the large ornamental wooden spoon from the kitchen. At some point, I drifted off, slipping just under the veil, not deep, restful sleep, superficial enough to be woken by the weakest of light energy reaching the West Coast. I rose, feeling unrested but ready to put that night behind me.

I'm not sure if you're aware, but routine can be a depressed person's friend and ally. Don't get me wrong, there is a sharp side to every two-edged sword, but having a routine, developing a "muscle memory" for activities that aren't preferred, can be a lifesaver. Do you ever have a hard time getting out of bed? The act of rising each morning can be one of the hardest things a sufferer has on their schedule. Prior to making a morning routine for myself, you couldn't believe the battles I fought just to put feet to floor. Depressed people hate beginnings, mostly because it means the beginning of having to go through stuff before we reach the end, which is our overarching goal, reach the end. Some mornings I was exhausted before I brushed my teeth. In 2011 I saw a movie that changed my life not because it was a great movie but because of the thirteen seconds it contained. The movie was *The Grey*, and if you're into wolf-on-human violence and freezing, it is a masterpiece. There was a spot in the movie where the protagonist, played by Liam Neeson, recalls his drunken, depressed poet father who wrote the following: "Once more into the fray, to the last good fight I will ever know. Live and die on this day. Live and die on this day."

I turned these twenty-six words into my morning mantra. As soon as my eyes open, I reach over and, with the push of a button, turn on the lamp next to the bed. My eyes squint from the instant bright harshness that assaults them. I lay back just long enough to recite my sacred incantation, swing my legs over the edge, and rise to my feet. I immediately make the bed. I take care to make it to meet

Lisa's exacting standards. This small routine is the absolute key to winning one of my hardest daily battles. "Once more into the fray," my mantra fixes my purpose with action. I don't have to succeed, I am not required to win, but I do have to fight; that is my steadfast requirement. I make the bed immediately and correctly, meaning that I take time to ensure the comforter is even on all sides and that the pillows are sufficiently fluffed and wrinkle-free, knowing that the better I make the bed, the less appealing the thought of making a hasty retreat will be.

Of course, it's earlier than most rise, but long after Lisa, who is out running, or biking, or swimming the English Channel. Years of working as a school bus driver have shaped her into a truly obnoxious morning person, one of those sick bastards who can rise with a smile and literally hit the ground running, without a mantra. Before meeting Lisa, I thought people like that were just an urban myth, like Chupacabra, tax refunds, or adult arcades having pinball machines.

You probably know someone who collects stuff. Some people collect stamps. Some people collect coins, art, or clipped toenails in a mason jar. We collect small furry rescue dogs who offensively demand a walk as soon as I'm physically able to. Izzi, the grande dame of the pack, came from the abusive neighbor of one of Lisa's coworkers. He would kick the small dog across his porch almost daily, much like Satan will to him when he's burning in hell if there is any justice. Hondo came to our family through an adoption event held at a local pet store where we were serendipitously dropping Izzi off for a grooming appointment. His name at the time was Wild Bill because of his unkempt hair and underbite, and he came from a puppy mill in San Jose where he had to fight for his food. In case you were wondering, I name my animals after characters in John Wayne movies, which is also how Maudie got her name (bonus points if you guess the movie). She came from our local humane society after I met her at a business presentation they had done for the Chamber of Commerce.

The only things that these three like more than a walk is pooping on the back patio and barking maniacally at every person or inanimate object that casts a shadow. I take them around the block like

I have for years, but every day is like their first, pulling and jumping and basically acting like little furry crackheads with a park-hopper pass to Crack-World, in Orlando. Their behavior is the number one reason I take them out as soon as I get up, before the "normal" people with their "normal" dogs make their daily circuit. Combined, my dogs weigh around twenty-five pounds, and I reason that if they were any bigger, they would be unwalkable, like tying three bottle rockets to strings, lighting them, and then taking a stroll. Walking my dogs is like volunteer charity work. It can be stressful or unpleasant, you may not really want to do it, but it's the right thing to do, and when you're done, you get a reward. That reward, for some, could be eternal life or a big tax write-off. For others, it may be a plaque on a bench. For me, it's coffee. Those first sips of hot dark-roast coffee in the morning feel like riding a dolphin while a strong gripped Swedish woman massages my back.

Normally I would take this moment to read the paper and get caught up on what's going on around town and around the world, but lately it's like taking a Xanax and reading the screenplay of *Schindler's List: The Musical.* I don't know how you process bad news, but here's the deal—you can't stick rainbow unicorns up your ass and pretend there aren't horrible parts of this world; there is no filter for the capacity of evil that people can bring to bear against other people. What you can do is limit your exposure, stop your paper, turn off the news, for fuck's sake get off social media, and focus on what you can control.

So now I sit with my mug of coffee and talk to you and work out my day. My focus now is getting stronger, taking the first working steps in taking on my PTSD, starting with fulfilling a commitment I made to Dr. K by calling to schedule two more sessions with her. After that, I will take a look at this breathing and meditation thing she spoke of. Personally, that "new-age, pan-flute-induced-feelings orgy" has never been my scene, but progress rarely happens inside your comfort zone or something I read on a poster, so check it out I will. For the first time I sense a change coming to my standard program of "moving forward at all costs" to "there is only one way out, and it is through." I firmly feel that the reason I am still alive is due to my ability to adapt and be proactive in the way I handle my depression. I have not always done it the right way, preferring to go around, over, or under often rather than through or head-on, but I always fought to make it to another day instead of killing my shadow by blocking out all light.

I went ahead a scheduled two more therapy sessions with Dr. K for July 9 and 23. I still feel the tug to self-sabotage or simply cancel the appointments and walk away feeling uncertain about a long process or doubting my ability to follow through. Do you realize how perfectly this illustrates how utterly frustrating the constant imbalance and conflict occurring between my ears can be? It's like a never-ending election year where one side's platform is progressive reform and positive change, and the other is committed to mayhem and destruction and wants nothing to change, ever, unless it's for the worse. Depression is an evil, manipulative, soul-sucking wraith, but I may have crossed a line there in comparing it to a politician running for office. I could say that for myself, and many sufferers would probably agree, we would be much better off without either.

Oh man, do you remember when I talked earlier about the ability to limit exposure to negative inputs where and when you can? Well, sometimes that is not possible; sometimes bad things happen when you're not ready for them. You can't avoid them, and they won't go away. Lisa just received a call from her mom, Nancy, letting us know that Bill, Lisa's stepfather is in the hospital with stage four cancer. My heart felt as if it had turned to iron in my chest. Poor Bill, fucking cancer. My thoughts immediately went to my mom, who lost her battle not long ago, and the emotional toll that it took on her and all our family. We knew that Bill had some health challenges lately, but we were totally unprepared for the severity of the diagnosis and prognosis.

Bill is a genuinely good guy who himself has overcome some serious personal demons to run a successful business before suffering a mental setback caused by anxiety and depression. He worked his way back from the brink, becoming a solid, stable, well-intentioned man. He is always there to help with a smile on his face. This news has hit me hard, at a time I am not ready to be hit hard. My depression is screaming in my ear, telling me to use this unfortunate news as an "out," to spin this into a viable excuse to not move forward with my therapy, to give up on the difficult sustained journey before it starts. It's this unconscionable bullshit that I need to kill. Do normal people have to deal with this? No, they don't, and I'm not going to either. I owe it to Bill to join his fight to survive by doing what I can for him and for myself. We will both rise to meet our enemy, we will both fight our fights and hope that fate is kind, and victory will be sweet. Those fights will happen, at least for now, three hours by car apart. COVID-19 precautions make it impossible to see Bill in the hospital and make the immediate trip south to visit and offer our love and support frustratingly pointless.

So today will end on a sour note. Many have ended this way. This is not new. The challenge will be tomorrow. How I deal with my depression is influenced heavily by momentum. I have often thought myself to be Sisyphus incarnate, the late son of Aeolus, whose ancient punishment for being an asshole was to push a large boulder up a hill, only to have it infuriatingly roll back down, over and over again. Like with most days of my life, the focus isn't in the victory. As much as I love a good victory, they are far too few and far between, making their absence an actual discouragement. Instead, I choose to focus on the fight, about pushing the stone as hard as I can no matter what altitude or lack thereof. I reach through my efforts. After a five-point-palm exploding heart-technique to the dick like Bill's diagnosis, that rock is going to feel like it's stuck in the mud, so I'm going to have to push extra hard tomorrow, which makes me hope tonight is large ornamental wooden spoon free.

THURSDAY, JUNE 25, 2020

I woke to an amazing cloudless summer morning. God's palette this morning was a lot of phthalo blue and alizarin crimson over a canvas prepared with liquid white. I had another restless night, too much seriousness, sometimes sleep can be a teasing little bitch. Speaking of little bitches, here's two woolly ones and a male one. What the hell is a male dog called? Regardless, they are expressing their desire to spread drops of urine in all the neighbor's groomed begonia beds. I get up and comply. My thoughts this morning over my cup of sacred brown bliss revolve around Bill and Nancy and what they must be going through this morning. There isn't anything more humbling than dealing with your own mortality or the potential loss of your best friend.

I'm sure that you've lost people. It's never easy, and no matter when it occurred, I'm sorry for your loss. My father officially died of an aortic aneurysm, but it was fucking cancer that ravaged his body in the months prior. Like Bill, my father's cancer started in his lungs and was a direct result of damage done by years of smoking. If you smoke, please stop. If not for your health, do it to just say "fuck you" to the tobacco companies that you are paying handsomely to drive your hearse to the cemetery. I was admonished from a very early age, "Don't ever smoke! It's a nasty habit," usually by my mother, often with a lit cigarette resting between her index and middle fingers. I complied not because she said not to, because I feel telling someone not to do something while you do it is dividing by zero, but because I could never fully understand the concept. You breathe smoke in just to expel it a moment later. I just don't get it, and don't get me started on fucking vaping. Are you a person or old-timey steam choo-choo?

While Bill was able to do what many can't, to quit, no matter how amazing of an accomplishment that is, it doesn't erase the damage already done. Neither of my parents was able to fully quit. They tried many, many times, but nicotine's grip on them proved just too mighty. They settled for cutting back and praying. My mother went from calling it her "nasty habit" to just her "nasty," which was the most unfortunate of word choices. There is nothing quite like finishing up a meal and having your mother declare, "I'm going to step out for a nasty." On a similar note, she would also, from time to time, forget where she stored her muscle massager and could be heard walking around her house asking, "Where is my vibrator? Have you seen my vibrator?"

My mom was a crazy lady and my biggest fan, no matter what stupid shit I would do or say. She also was the most faithful person I have ever met. She believed in God's plan and walked her belief every day, so when she was diagnosed with terminal fucking cancer almost two years ago, she was already at peace. I wasn't with her when she passed, I had a work conference in Atlanta, and almost as soon as I landed, her health started to take a turn for the worse. I rebooked my flight but couldn't get out until the first flight the following morning. She passed when I was on final approach to Salt Lake City, my connection home. Every once in a blue moon, you meet a beautiful soul, seemingly too good to be walking among us dirty sinners. My mom was one. Noah was one. I'm not. Dr. K touched briefly on my comments about my mom's passing by asking if I had come to peace and closure with her death. I told her that I had not. I move forward at all costs, or at least I used to, so I will definitely have some reckoning to do at some point soon, but not today.

Okay, I've decided to talk with you on a daily basis about things I'm going through or have gone through, with the hopes of increasing a better understanding of a life lived with depression, with the hopes that perhaps it could be of at least a slight benefit to someone else who suffers. I feel that it's time to bring some of these things to light, and I feel that we've developed enough of a rapport that the things

I tell you will be kept in context to the bigger issues of depression and its impacts. Don't worry, I won't make it weird and talk about my freezer filled with body parts or my closet full of leather whips and ass-less chaps. Wait, aren't all chaps ass-less? I don't know cowboy stuff. I just want to give an honest, transparent attempt to illustrate how depression has disturbed my life and what I've done about that disturbance. Now that we've reached a level of understanding in our relationship, let's move forward.

I think that I've talked about plumbing before, it's a big issue with me, and we're about to get into it, but first I need to talk with you cursing because these topics go together like bathtubs and toasters. You have probably already guessed that I will use colorful language from time to time based on the perceived appropriateness of the situation. I see cursing as a lifestyle choice that aligns with my core values. I don't know exactly what that means, but it sounds official. If you are easily upset or if you are offended by something, or everything, that I've said, I would probably look for alternative reading material because I'm going to say what's on my mind per our agreement, and some of it is going to be crazy shit. Now I try to keep a level of propriety and decorum in my behavior, so I stay somewhere on the vulgarity scale between Mr. Rodgers stubbing his toe and the crazy meth fiend on the corner screaming obscenities at a stuffed elephant with its plastic eye dangling precariously on its side. That being said, when I walked into the bathroom and saw the sink clogged with shaving cream and dark water, I channeled my inner Samuel L. Jackson. "What the fuck. Who the fuck clogged the fucking sink? Someone needs to take one of those fucking snakes off the fucking plane and use it to unclog the fucking sink!"

I had it in my head that it was our oldest son, Mack, who has been living with us since being honorably discharged from the US Army. The plan was to stay with us while he finished his schooling and pilot training, working toward his plans of becoming a professional flyer. As with most best-laid plans, Mack's course heading altered with time and circumstance. He is now close to finalizing a job in the law enforcement field, which may come in handy down the road. We have always told him our house will always be his home, but the more time passes, the more that statement reads like a question. It turns out it was Noah who was the perpetrator of the offensive clog, and he was very sorry. Being mad at Noah is like punching baby Yoda in the face, and nothing makes Noah happier than when he is able to do tasks that make him feel more independent, like shaving. So now I'm a dick with a clogged sink.

Why plumbing? Why do I have such deep-rooted psychological entanglements with one of the marvels of the modern world? That is an excellent question. I'm glad you asked it. Like most complex neurotically fabricated "strandbeest," the original blueprints of my plumbing issues trace their beginnings to my childhood. Over the years, I have amended the design and added little ticks and neurosis to it until it is now this monstrous clogged, dripping, emotional mess that I try to kill with Liquid Plumber.

I have never in my life lived in a new home. I have never lived in a quasi-new home, unless you are talking geologically. Don't get me wrong, I have lived in great houses filled with love and waffles, but they were all old. To hear my father speak of the house I grew up in was to hear a story of a horse pasture with a shack made of papier-mache and hard biscuits. Working together, he and my mom built the house and cultivated the land to make a home. My dad worked in insurance and investments. He wasn't a carpenter by trade and definitely not a plumber. Don't get me wrong, the dude could make it work; he was a maker, a scholar, an artist, a true renaissance man, just not a plumber. He was constantly under a sink, scraping his knuckles, saying "Shit!" or "Dammit!" never in my recollection using my go-to imprecation, "Fuck." My experience is that if you don't say "Fuck" when you plumb, you probably never will.

My dad was a caring, nurturing soul who never raised his hands to his children and was slow to raise his voice in anger, at least to his children. To others he would be happy to give a thundering rebuke. The rare occasion when you did find yourself on the wrong side of his graces, you remembered it. He had a thing about shower curtains. You should always ensure that they are pressed against the tub enclosure to prevent water from escaping down the side of the tub and pooling on the floor. After one long, distracted shower, where I sang

"Physical" by Olivia Newton John instead of washing or ensuring the shower curtain was firmly pressed against the tub enclosure, he entered the bathroom and pointed directly to the puddle formed on the bathroom floor, a crazed look in his eye, as if I had just slapped him with wet teenage underwear. Now he may have been agitated by having to wait. Living in a one-bathroom house meant having to plan ahead, but when words came out of his mouth, they did so with intention and energy, "Do you see this! This right here! This water is right now, as we speak, seeping down between the tub and the floor and is rotting our house from underneath us!" He would always tell me that someday I would understand, and he was absolutely right.

Not only do I understand, I have tried to instill in my family the importance of shower curtain discipline and how our house is slowly dissolving around us. My children do not understand, and I fear the family plumbing psychosis may be coming to an end, despite my best attempts to instill in them an almost paranormal understanding and respect. They just don't seem to care enough to stay up at night wondering when they would end up in the bottom of an enormous sinkhole crater caused by slipshod shower curtain protocols.

Do you know that plumbing is about much more than pipes or fittings? Plumbing is about control, the ability to master our surroundings and create function and harmony. When there is a dripping faucet, you have lost that control, and with every *ploop* an impacting water droplet makes as it collides with the hard porcelain sink, it reminds you of that. Soon the *ploop*s get louder, more aggressive and annoying until it reaches "soccer commentator" level, but instead of riotously yelling "Goal!" all I hear is "Ploop!" every eight seconds. If you have depression, then you know how important control is. I think it's important to make a distinction at this point. Control does not mean manipulation. I do not attempt, nor obviously would I be very good at, bending people to my will or by force of coercion or intimidation dictating thoughts, feelings, or actions. Control equals predictability, and predictability equals stability. Control is a warm blanket on a cool night. It is a sense of security that our depression cannot prey on, that it can't use against us. Control is a weapon or a threat, depending on what side of the trigger you're on, so not having it in areas of your life like relationships and finances can be a real liability.

I know that there's a question you have been patiently waiting to ask, and I'm about to answer it. Why don't I just hire a plumber? The answer is closely tied to control and finances and, yes, some level of insecurity. I think that I've mentioned to you that my house is sixty-four years old, with pipes that were installed when Dwight D. Eisenhower was in the Oval Office. My entire plumbing system is held together with duct tape, plumber's putty, and positive vibes, so it is entirely within the scope of believability that a twelve-cent leaking gasket could end up costing me sixteen thousand dollars, which makes my asshole pucker.

I know a lot of people in a lot of professions. Do you need a good lawyer or banker? I got you covered. Are you looking for barbequed squirrel meat? I got a squirrel guy. What I don't have in my junk drawer next to the batteries with dubious levels of charge is a business card for a plumber whom I know and trust. I know, back to the control thing, but being bent over a financial barrel is not a position that fills me with joy, and having someone hold the financial upper hand in a captive relationship when I don't even have a coupon or Groupon sucks ballcock. My transactions with plumbers are reminiscent of the scene in *National Lampoon's Vacation*, where Clark drives off the road in the middle of nowhere, then wanders the desert looking for help before reuniting with his family at a dilapidated gas station.

When asking the charcoal-sketchy attendant how much repairs cost, he is told, "How much you got?"

"No, seriously, how much are the repairs?"

The ragged, unscrupulous man slaps a box-end wrench into his open hand, leans toward Clark, and says, "All of it, boy!"

I know, it sounds like I've just offended the very people who hold the ability to fix my biggest non-brainal problem, but my issue isn't with plumbers who are honest, hardworking people, but with my issue of lack of institutional control over the scope of the problem area, which, the way I see it, is plumbing.

Speaking of issues, I'm not actually done. If that wasn't enough baggage crammed underneath the sink cupboards and between the crawlspace joists, I have also glued my fear of failure and, to a minor degree, my self-worth to plumbing. I know that you've seen all the cheesy motivational posters about failure, like it's an essential part of success or that the only real failure is not trying. You can shine that turd, but failure is failure. I get that you grow wiser and more resolute through the experience, but you have failed, and with that comes consequence. Pain and failure have been my YouTube since when it was MeTube and consisted of perpetual inter-brainal replays of my deficiencies.

I absolutely get that nobody likes to fail. Every time Edison failed at the lightbulb, he would strip to his boxers, curl up into a ball, and let small goats climb all over him. I know you know this, but I'm going to say it anyway. The pressure we feel is 100 percent self-imposed. We put pressure on ourselves to provide for our families, we take our responsibilities seriously, we try to live up to standards provided to us, so when we fail, we feel that we have failed more than ourselves, and we have failed those around us and those who came before us. Of course, this is all bullshit, but it doesn't change the fact that it exists, and it plays absolute havoc with depression. My depression absolutely loves when I get mental about pipes and leaks and gains strength when I fail because of the psychological fallout that is sure to follow, and I know it has an outright boner when I allow failure to lower my self-worth.

You see, when it comes to depressive disorder, insecurities can abound and prove deadly. For me, plumbing isn't just plumbing. I think that you see that picture a little more clearly now, but for others, it may be familial relationships, or weight or health concerns, or even sexual freakery. If you are a sufferer, be aware of your vulnerabilities, know how they affect you, and talk about it to those who are close to you. It will possibly explain some erratic behavior and strengthen the relationship, not weaken your value. If you know or love a sufferer, be aware that there are forces at play that you are not aware of, and be patient and supportive. It may at the moment seem insignificant to you, but it is very real to us.

It's amazing the things that depressed people can attach emotional baggage to. It can be practically anything real or imaginary. Emotive weight can be put behind people, places, or things that carry importance and positive, or negative, significance in our lives, and once depression interweaves itself throughout the psychological strata of that issue, there is no possible way to separate it. One day I will have my old pipes replaced with new, and my depression will have one less issue to hold over my head. Until then, I think I'll close out today with a quote from Albert Einstein, who once said, "If I had my life to live over again, I'd be a plumber." The more I think about it, maybe I would too.

FRIDAY, JUNE 26, 2020

"People, people who need people are the luckiest people in the world," I hate that fucking song. It's so slow. I don't remember when it came out or who sung it, but I remember that line, and while I haven't always believed in its message, I do now. At one dark point in my life, I just wanted to walk off alone into the sunset, become a pack of one, and wander the desert kicking random people in the face like Lone Wolf McQuade. The problem with that is that most people aren't wired for social isolation. We actually require human touch and connection and, without it, commence a slow trudge toward madness. Never forget the harrowing adventures of Tom Hanks in *Castaway*, where FedEx shipped him to a deserted isle, and in isolation, he befriended a volleyball named Wilson, who became his friend and confidant, until Wilson slept with Lola, the coconut Hanks had his eye on, so he drowned him and set him adrift. I'm not kidding. Loneliness will mess with your mind.

The dark irony when you live with depression is that, while you still need human interaction, you want to withdraw rather than engage and would rather remain silent than communicate. This is often aggravated by our inability to describe what we are experiencing internally. It is so hard to describe how we are feeling, and that difficulty generates a short circuit somewhere between our brain and mouth. From there, the meaning gets lost, the words get jumbled around, and what comes out sounds a lot like "I'm fine." The depression playbook is heavy with how to go through your day, appearing normal for all intents and purposes, without actually saying anything of substance or having any kind of meaningful interactions

33

with other humans. Back in the day, I could go weeks appearing like a functioning member of society, and that's when I was married and had kids, ran a business, and did volunteer stuff. I showed up, I worked, and when I got tired of telling people I was "fine," I would tell them I was "good," and while they may not have believed me, nobody pushed the issue.

The older I get, the more value and benefit I receive from being around the human spirit. I have found benefit in what others bring to my life and have appreciated the diverse opportunities to increase my own humanity through others that I would have never been open to when I was a younger man. Communication is unquestionably fundamental to not only depression management, but to your relationships, your growth and understanding, and to a great degree, your quality of life. I don't tell people what to do. Wait a minute, I always tell people what to do, but I don't expect them to listen. That being said, if I had to give just one piece of advice to someone who I imagine doesn't have time for two pieces of advice, I would tell them, just talk. Talk about sports or weather, talk about that time you kissed your cousin behind the boatshed for five bucks and some Necco wafers if you want to. Just know this, if you can talk about something, you can talk about everything.

This is such a change for me since my younger days. If Lisa had to tell you what the hardest part of living with a depressive is, she would say my penis. I apologize for that. Sometimes I can't resist my urges to turn into a teenage dipshit, and she would never say anything that would encourage that behavior. What she would say 100 percent of the time she would be asked that question is communication difficulties. It's so hard to be a couple when you're not only not on the same page; you're not even in the same library. I made her feel isolated and alone. In essence, when I was withdrawing, I was doing it for both of us. A part of me actually believed that I was doing it altruistically, that my emotional abandonment was actually saving her from experiencing my darkness, when in reality, I was condemning her to her own.

I know that you're a great listener. You've shown that, but how at you at talking? Maybe you're a great communicator but are with someone who isn't. That's the absolute pisser, isn't it? You can be Oprah, but your success as a conversationalist is reliant on the willingness and ability of at least one other person. Like I said, if you can talk about something, you can talk about anything, but sometimes it's the first words, where awkwardness needs to be overcome and comfort established, that are the most crucial. If someone is suffering from PTSD or has experienced physical or emotional trauma, you will probably want to start with something way more comfortable like the impact the early Mongol Empire had on Western civilization or the size of walrus dicks. There is magic, believe me, in sharing time and words with others, even more when it's over a cup of steamy, imported bean water brewed to perfection.

Today I needed to be around people, I think everyone who has "sheltered in place" due to the coronavirus has a newfound appreciation for the freedoms we all enjoy and take for granted, so since I can, I head to my favorite coffee shop. I ordered my usual, the drip, scalding hot water over finely ground beans, coffee the way goddess Caffeina intended it. I secretly hope every time that the barista completes my order, they ask aloud, "Who's the drip?" just so I can proudly say, "I am, I'm the drip." It always seemed way funnier in my head. I wonder why because that sucked. Anyway, Noah, who would go to a tax audit to get out of the house, joined me and ordered his favorite blended dessert in a cup with a tablespoon of coffee to make it legit, and we sat down. It wasn't long until we were joined by a couple of folks that I know from business networking meetings before they were replaced by the now infamous Brady Bunch-esque group, Zoom. Oh, how I have missed people's energy and divergent points of view. I sit and write words while others communicate with their worlds via phone or tablet. This is not the Algonquin Round Table or Mission Command, but today it feels absolutely like a hub of activity, like business is being done and movement is building toward momentum.

Over the hour we sat, the topics of discussion didn't wander far from what we had been dealing with personally and professionally since March, taking time, of course, to solve all of the world's problems in case someone asks, but they won't. I asked those assembled about their thoughts or experiences with mindfulness or meditation. Given the personality of this crew, I wasn't expecting much and was neither surprised nor disappointed. I let the topic die a quiet death and made a note to do some research on the shiny Google box later. Noah was long done with his drink and was bowling on his tablet; every once in a while I would hear him get a strike. My coffee cup was light in my hand, so I gave it one last swirl and gulp, and we said our goodbyes and headed toward my office.

I used to go to the office every day whether I had to be there for meetings or not, preferring to keep a firm separation between work and not work. I felt that without firm boundaries, I was far too prone to distraction, which I would "look at the size of that fucking tractor! Why would anyone need a tractor that big, really?" When the pandemic hit and overnight all meetings and events were canceled, I shifted to working mostly from home. Given the technology available, it wasn't hard to do, and I have found that I could actually get more done if I work all day, not just eight hours of it. If I had known this thirty years ago, I could be ruling the world, or at least be successful enough to own a racehorse named Deez Hors Nutz, and I would charge a ton for his sperm.

Dr. K, at the conclusion of our therapy session, assigned me some homework that I have not yet begun, which historically is par for the course. She asked that I check out mindfulness, breathing exercises, and meditation, and I reluctantly agreed. I say reluctant because in my mind, I see various crystals and a patchouli-drenched, under-groomed hippie lighting an incense stick that is actually labeled "unfortunate body odor." Yes, you are absolutely correct. I have been called closed-minded and at times have indeed been made uncomfortable by women with armpit hair, but I feel that progress is being made in this area. So here I am downloading an app on my phone called Calm. I don't hold great expectations in this arena, for over five decades I have shown no abilities or talent for any discipline requiring the focus of attention. When I was in church as a child, adolescent, and honestly, adult, and the grand potentate would tell his flock to close their eyes, focus their thoughts, and lift their prayers to the Almighty, I was wondering why the fuck the Hamburglar didn't just eat Officer Big Mac. I mean, he's a hamburger. Regardless, I chose Calm because I saw an advertisement on the television that said "do nothing for thirty seconds," and I'm like, "I think I can make that happen."

So it turns out the daily sessions are around ten minutes in length, so immediately I'm thinking that there's no way that I'm going to get this brain to slow down and focus for five whole minutes, let alone ten, but as the poster in the breakroom next to the sign forbidding the microwaving of fish products says, "Growth starts where your comfort zone ends." Feeling immediate motivation, I click on the new tile on my phone screen and get ready to open my mind to new possibilities.

Do you know what I hate? Not enough choices. Do you know what I hate more? Too many choices. It's the Netflix conundrum. If I want to watch something at seven o'clock, I have to start down that rabbit hole no later than quarter after six, and even then I just don't know if I want to commit to that genre or go documentary. I'm immediately surprised by the depth and breadth of the meditation and relaxation options laid out before me. I can literally stay in a catatonic state until International "Everything You Think Is Wrong" Day, which, as it happens, is March 15, unless you're unsure if that is correct. It's like standing in the supermarket staring at a wall of wieners trying to figure out which package will best fulfill my needs while a virtual carousel of glittery meat tubes spins around my head. Just when I was about to click off the app and play Bubble Pop, I ran across an option called "the daily calm," giddyap.

I put my AirPods in, "wrong ears again, Voltaire," then I put them in the correct ears and hit play. Actually I just pushed the picture. There was no actual play button, just for your personal information, in case you were looking for a play button. I was immediately greeted by a woman's voice that draped my ears with velvety fleece and made me feel immediately at ease. She told me how to sit, how to hold my hands, how to breathe. She told me how to focus and how it's all right if I lose it, because I can find it again, then after a few minutes of allowing me to play "tag" with my inner brain, she told me a story about a lake and the importance of being present.

Then it was over. Ten minutes had passed quickly, effortlessly. I felt good, a little accomplished. Of course, the next thing to do is to contemplate, to understand how what I just learned can fit into my life, where I can grow. I like how I feel, it's hard to explain, but I feel refreshed, like I took a nap, but without the nap hangover you get sometimes when you wake up foggy, like you need a nap. I click off and then go immediately to Bubble Pop, fucking level 212. I can't seem to get close, but maybe now that I'm focused.

As much as I enjoyed my mini-mental spa day, I don't know how this event will play into my depression issues. I can definitely feel an increase in my calmness, which is truth in advertising. I'll at the very least give them that much. All in all, it was an eye-opener for my first experience. I went into it with an open mind and was rewarded by an experience that surpassed my expectations. I would love it if this turned into a viable weapon against my depression, and the irony would be delicious, using peace and calm to defeat a dark evil, yummy.

Saturday, June 27, 2020

Saturdays have always had their own rhythm around our house that closely matches the rhythm of most Mondays through most Fridays. Lisa, per usual, is the alarm clock and, per usual, is up twenty minutes earlier than I would prefer. Our lives are built around structure, routine, and discipline, which offers stability and builds mental toughness and endurance. This regimen will come in handy when society breaks down, and all we will have standing between the ravenous hordes of barbaric neomodern Neanderthals and our protein powder and fennel seeds is our wits, endurance, and small spears fashioned from stool legs.

Things happen pretty fast in the morning, not a lot of downtime, which is diametrically opposite of my childhood that consisted of cereal, cartoons, and nothing else until grown-up programming took over on all three channels. First thing Lisa and I will do is writhe around getting sweaty, listening to music that is way younger than our demographic. We work out together as much as our schedule allows, which has been almost daily since the ankle-monitor-less house arrest began in March. I'm a big believer in exercise as a management tool for depression and will undoubtedly go into more on this at some point, but I have a bunch on my mind today that I need to talk about. This is the day, one week removed, that I lost my shit, experienced what PTSD feels like, and nearly suffered a catastrophic defeat at the hands of my sworn enema. I know I said *enema*. It was a dig at my depression. It hates when I call him that. Nevertheless, here's what's on the schedule. Joshua is due for a visit later, and my under bathroom sink plumbing is still being held together by rubber bands and the "light" side of the force, so it's safe to say that I'm freaking out a little.

Before I can freak out more, however, coffee, then grocery shopping. My first cup I take at the kitchen table as a victory lap for not stroking out during a grueling workout, which I feel gets likelier every day. The coffee today is a dark South American variety that has a smoky flavor with nutty highlights that makes me slightly euphoric as the aroma enters my nostrils. I sit relaxed, close my eyes, and spend a minute doing a focused breathing exercise from yesterday. I feel like a kid with a new toy who just wanted to make sure it still worked, and sure enough, I'm able to wrangle the greased pig that is my conscious mind. I feel the same freshness around my senses as I take another sip, and use it to adjust my attitude, set my intentions, and get my head about my day. I pour what coffee I have remaining into a travel mug, being sure not to waste a drop, fill it up with fresh, grab Noah, and head to the grocery store.

Are you a good shopper? What I mean is, do you like looking for deals, checking prices or ingredients, cutting coupons, comparing brands? I fucking hate it. I'm not a good shopper. I always feel like there is something better I could be doing with my time, like hooking a rubber band around my pinkie, wrapping it around my thumb, and resting the other loop end across my pointer finger like a gun, then shooting stuff, and people, or dogs. I make big decisions every day and do it with confidence and a high degree of ability, but if you only write ketchup on a shopping list, I'm going to stare at three hundred different goddamn bottles for what seems like way longer than a grown man should until I grab one. Then I look at it, then I look back at the others. Do I go with my first gut reaction, or do I make a change? It's like a Scantron test in school without the number two pencils or the odor. Next on the list salad dressing, son of a bitch!

We work up and down the aisles, making sure to check the list, which really is just a picture I took of the list on my phone, so I didn't have to bring the list, because somewhere in my mind's eye, it seemed like the most efficacious use of my time. I'll tell you one thing I loathe in this life, and that's backtracking. I can't stand going backward to go forward. It cuts across my grain like few things, so I take special care not to overlook listed items. I have been known to simply leave said list entries behind, preferring to tell Lisa they were out than to retrace my steps.

"Hmm, the grocery store was out of bread?"

"Yeah, it was the damnedest thing, there must be some kind of shortage, people using it for toilet paper or something."

I will also look at what other people have in their carts and will silently judge them for their choices. Don't tell me you've never passed someone with a cart full of chips, Twinkies, and beer and thought, "You may want to add some toilet paper to your order while you're here." Just don't get caught looking because people get huffy and weird.

Having fewer people is a definite advantage to shopping early Saturday, and since we shop practically every week, it cuts way down on planning. Our list, in fact, is basically stuff we ran out of, for the other stuff we need, we are reliant on our memory. Mealtime around our house is different than most, I believe. We don't plan big elaborate dinners with an entrée and a couple of sides, and we pass them around the table and smile at each other. At our house, it's kinda like a buffet where each person picks a couple of things to eat, then that person cooks them and eats them, no pomp or circumstance. Most nights we all eat different meals, but we eat together, we share a mealtime, and that is an important time together. Sometimes we think we need things every week when we actually don't, so it's not uncommon for our pantry to have a much greater percentage of dill pickles and instant pudding than most people's should. I sense you silently judging me, and that's all right.

Noah loves to be independent. We use this time at the grocery store to build on that independence by talking to him about meal planning and ingredients. He loves to cook his own meals, and by shopping, he is learning how to better take care of himself and advocate for the things that he enjoys. Before he was rendered nonessential by the restaurant where he worked as a kitchen helper, Noah would also get a real kick of paying for his groceries as well, which also made me feel good that I didn't have to. But for now, we take it one day at a time and head to the self-checkout, where we scan and bag our own groceries. Today Noah's job will be scanning, and I will take the bagger job, which means if the milk's on the eggs, it's on my watch. I'm generally a man who knows his strengths and limitations, but I tell you this unreservedly, I am probably the best bagger around. Years of playing Tetris has trained me well, so as Noah deftly scans each item and hands them to me, I'm running the volume calculations in my head and putting them in the appropriate void. I have four bags going at once. You can play chess all you want. This here is a real-world skill honed in the virtual world. Just wait until the earth is surrounded by menacing asteroids; get me a spaceship with blasters and a booster, grab a beer, and watch the show.

We have a galley kitchen that was made for hobbits, or maybe sixty-four years ago, people were generally smaller. Regardless, when any activity requires more than one person in the kitchen at any given time, choreography and patience are required. Lisa handles the cold stuff, getting the freezer and fridge organized as she puts the new purchases away, carefully, deliberately. I put the dry pantry goods away with far less care, like an impudent child forced to put his toys away before he gets a massage, or a hundred dollars, or whatever parents bribe their kids with nowadays.

As the sun crosses the sky, my thoughts increasingly turn to Josh's upcoming visit. A nervous anticipation starts to build. It's a hell of a thing to be afraid of your own son, it's unnatural and uncomfortable, and I want it to stop. My mind rests on what Dr. K said to me: "PTSD is just thoughts" and "If it bleeds, we can kill it." The second quote was actually from the movie *Predator*, but I think the intention is the same. I reason that if PTSD is indeed just thoughts, and we learn how to control our thoughts, then we can control our PTSD. Of course, this is a gross oversimplification of an arduous process that will undoubtedly take real time and effort to accomplish, but there is logic to it.

I'm not going to lie to you. There was a time when claiming PTSD was such an avant-garde thing to do that I questioned the veracity of some people's claims. I never questioned a veteran's claims, especially a combat veteran. If they tell me the earth is flat, I will believe them. They have earned that. By the way, if anyone else says the earth is flat, I will tell them that they are single-handedly lowering the bar for all of humanity, even stupid humanity. The person I'm talking about is the bleach blonde glittered floof bomb talking to her friend Amythasia in line at Starbucks. "Oh my God. I'm having PTSD from the last time I was here. They replaced my 148-degree Brazil nut milk with soy, and I thought I was going to die." I can tell you, now from experience, that PTSD is not a bad memory. It is a physical assault on your body and your senses and is no fucking joke. I have a newfound appreciation and respect for those who have genuinely suffered.

PTSD may be thoughts, but your brain doesn't know that, so connecting my conscious to my subconscious is going to buy my immediate challenge. I must be proactive, mindful in my approach, and diligent in my effort. I must think every day and use meditation and contemplation as tools. I will overcome this misfortune because the alternative is unacceptable. I am still alive because I am resolute in my desire to not give in to my depression. Every day that I am above ground is in spite of its best effort to the contrary. Do not underestimate the lengths I will go if you make me dig in my heels. I will not hesitate to cancel a picnic.

I don't know, from a psychological point of view, if it's an advantage or disadvantage that I spend time weekly with the person who is the root cause of my PTSD. I know that sounds can be powerful triggers. Sudden loud noises or angry guttural verbalizations like he would use prior to an aggression always get my attention. The challenge is that he makes similar noises when he's happy or excited, or maybe a little mad, so this afternoon may be very interesting, like taking long drives with gangsters and cannolis, interesting.

When J Man arrives, he is greeted with a kiss and a drink that we make up that is spiked with some CBD. I'm a big fan of "the devil's dandelions." Marijuana has been a legal substance in our state for a couple of years now, and I will use it recreationally, like my kayak. I don't smoke marijuana believing in not smoking anything but meat, and for the sake of transparency, I feel like I should say that I personally don't own a smoker or the time or understanding to use it, but I like meat, especially the meat with meat in it. Josh's dosage comes from a tincture made of the plants' oil as does the edible gummies that I take from time to time, especially if I need a little help sleeping, which lately has been often.

The first time ever that I sampled marijuana was years ago when we were interested in seeing how Josh would react to it, whether it would affect his mood or behavior. A pothead friend with vast experience and smelly clothes provided us with spiked cookies for when Josh next visited. Having no prior experience of frame of reference, Lisa and I decided to eat a cookie, akin to the royal food tasters of old. It wasn't until later that we found out that a normal dose would have been a quarter of a cookie. Another interesting fact we were unaware of is that there is an activation period for edible marijuana products, meaning it has to go through your digestive system before you feel it, anywhere from forty-five minutes to an hour and a half. We went from thinking that smelly hippie ripped us off to thinking that we had just checked into Dr. Frank-N-Furter's castle on Halloween. Lisa was composing an email when it hit her. She was unable to write the word "then," she physically and mentally couldn't do it, and it freaked her out. I couldn't either but mostly because I was laughing so hard tears were streaming down my face. The world had become an episode of *Benny Hill*, and I loved it. Lisa, on the other hand, not so much. She was convinced she was going to jail. At one point hearing sirens in the distance, she hid in our closet.

The effects lasted a few really weird hours, but in the end, the high wore off with no lingering side effects or hangover, so we decided that a normal dose would be safe to try on Josh, and the experiment was a success. It mellowed the big man out, it gave him the munchies like a wet gremlin, but he was chill. Now it's just a routine thing that happens when he comes over. He gets his "reefer colada," heads to his room, takes off his clothes, and plops on the bed. Like when he was living with us, Lisa and I rotate who's on point, meaning someone has always got to be in charge and aware of what the big guy is up to. When you're on point, you have "the con." The ship, or starship, is under your control, and the other can do chores, watch something on TV, or shave the hair off a llama. We pass control back and forth as required and like a choreographed well-oiled machine designed to oil other machines.

The time passed rather quickly and without incident, and while I never achieved a level of comfort or relaxation during the visit, I likewise never dissolved into a quivering puddle of saliva with testicles. Like most weeks, Josh decided he wanted to eat everything in the house that didn't have a heartbeat and would intently seek food, but he did not get agitated when we "cut him off." Just to be safe, however, we hid the dogs. Big J spent some time shredding, which is a preferred activity and is exactly like it sounds. He will take cardboard or foam, sometimes fabric or wood, and rip it up into tiny pieces with his fingers and, now and again, his teeth. He stands in his bathroom and throws the fragments out the window, through the screen that he ripped out. We put a bucket out there to catch some of it, but weekly cleanup is often required. Over the years, he has shredded some stuff we'd rather of stayed unshredded, like family pictures, my paintings, money, and Randy "Macho Man" Savage's autograph. Needless to say, we try and monitor what he has access to, but for a huge man, he can be sneaky.

Lisa always likes to get him cleaned up before taking him back to his house. She is an amazing mother who believes there's no excuse for not leaving the house looking and smelling good, and she wants both for him when he leaves us. As big as Josh is, he requires help with most of the acts of daily living, such as bathing, so she'll get him in the shower and start straightening his room. Josh loves a shower. He can stay in there being soothed by the hot water for quite a while. My lowest point as a father happened twelve or thirteen years ago when I started a shower for J, checked the temperature, made sure it was perfect, got him undressed and in, sprayed him down, and then got busy and totally forgot about him. I don't remember exactly how long I left him, long enough to hurt my heart, long enough to hurt my heart twelve or thirteen years later. He emerged from the ordeal a little pruny, but none the worse for wear and absolutely squeaky clean.

I help load our big man into Lisa's car. He smells fresh and clean. I give him a kiss on the cheek and tell him I love him and that

I'm proud of him, buckle his seatbelt, and shut his door. I am always torn when he drives away, but especially today. I know at some point I'm going to have to open the box, the one with the "never fucking open" sign nailed on it, where I stuff all of my guilt issues, but I'm not going there right now. Today, like most weeks, I feel relief when he leaves, and I hate myself for it, but still it's there. The relief I feel is compounded by the fact that I didn't have a PTSD episode, that the running water worked, and the concern about a repeat of last week was unfounded. I often dreamed of a "normal" life, where I could spend time with my family without fear, where we could talk and I could share my experience and help them build a life, that I wasn't filled with angst or absolution at their coming and going. A "normal" life, it seems, was never in the cards, so I can cry about a rigged deck and feel sorry for myself, or I can appreciate the gifts given that may be overlooked if everything had gone to plan. I once read a quote from Maya Angelou on a card or something that said, "If you are always trying to be NORMAL, you will never know how AMAZING you can be." Now that's some feel-good shit that's on point. Time to go be amazing.

Do you enjoy Sundays? It's been my experience that most people do. For me, Sundays have been one of my least favorite days of the week, going way back to my childhood. For this, I blame several things that most people hold dear, so bear with me. We may part company on some of my viewpoints, but that doesn't mean I'm right or that you're wrong. I'm just working the process trying to do this transparency thing, and that means getting it all out there, so here we go. It is my personal belief that I would have a much different relationship with Sunday if it wasn't for Mondays, the church, or the NFL.

Whatever your views of Mondays are, I'm sure that you will agree that often the malevolent nature of an upcoming Monday will cast a long shadow that darkens the preceding Sunday. It may be a big assignment or a report due. It may just be the start of another trudging week, but more beautiful Sunday afternoons have been ruined by the dark specter of approaching doom than I care to think about. Now I know that point of view and attitude play a large role in thoughts and feelings, but in the depressed community, Monday is just the worst. Monday signifies a new beginning, a fresh slate for the week, which, for people who don't suffer, could be a good constructive thing, but for those of us who do, it means enduring another week of darkness and uncertainty. When you wear a mask every day, not the mask to keep your bacteria, mucus, and dead cells from flying all over people's faces when you talk to them, but the mask that shows people that you're "fine," it gets exhausting, and Mondays are especially dubious since, for most of us, it signifies another long week of mask wearing.

The problem is that Monday is more of a state of mind than an actual day. If you say "Fuck it, I no longer will work Mondays," and you're lucky enough to be in a position to do so, then Tuesday will become your Monday, and nothing, in essence, would have changed. Tuesday would pick up the mantle as Sith lord and mind-choke the hell out of Monday, rendering it subservient and less favorable. No matter what weekday begins your workweek, it is always your Monday, just as the end is your Friday. It just so happened for me, most of my life Monday was on Monday, and Sunday suffered for it. I can't tell you how many times I've been told to "suck it up" or given some bullshit motivation about attitude, and every time, it makes me smile. The person probably thinks that they did me a profound service, that I'm smiling because they filled me with a newfound energy from the significance of their pep talk. They don't realize that the smile is a result of my mental image of wrapping my Italo Ferretti silk tie that I never wear around their throat and, with gentle pressure, choking them out. Depression does not equal lazy. It does not indicate a lack of ability or motivation. If you had to struggle every day to put one fucking foot in front of the next, fight hard to maintain a job and a life, trade every iota of strength for some small degree of normalcy, then maybe you'd not be as thrilled to see another week start so goddamn soon.

Something you should understand before we go forward is that I have made it a point in my life to never talk about religion or politics since it turns many functioning, respectful adults into raging whack-job assholes. I'm going to break that rule for you because I feel that religion is a big piece of my depression puzzle, and if we want the full picture, we have to show all the pieces. My view on politics doesn't really factor because I feel that all politics and political issues are the same, fucking Nazis prying open the ark of the covenant; the only way to get out alive is to close your eyes and act like it isn't happening.

Before I ever experienced depression, back when life was pure and carefree, church was just an inconvenience, a place I had to put pants on for in-between Sunday comics and Sunday breakfast, which was the best. I remember having to go to children's church, which I disliked because I wasn't able to fart out loud. I do remember hearing the Bible stories and being taught how to pray. Even then I couldn't focus for very long. I hope it's link sausage this morning and not that spicy patty sausage. From an early age, it seemed to me that there was only one accepted way to do things, one way to pray, to act, and to treat others, and it was a way that never came naturally to me, but being the respectful child, I went without complaint and sat there, unfarting.

Things took a turn for me religiously when I was thirteen and met the devil. Armed with the vast repertoire of theological knowledge that I had gleaned between daydreams, I was certain that I was indeed facing something evil, and I'd learned enough that when you confront evil, you pray to God with all of your heart, soul, and ability. I'm fucked. I didn't really know how to pray, and yes, I know now God understands all, and in reality, there are many ways to pray, but I was thirteen and also believed eating a watermelon seed would grow a watermelon inside me that I would have to poop out.

Those early days of my depression were hard, especially since making the decision to not tell my parents. A decision shaped by two things: the church and my uncle Jack, who was living at our house at the time. Jack Deevers was a Vietnam veteran who never found purpose in his life. He was a bipolar (manic-depressive), like a lot of the apples off my father's family tree, who would go off his meds at the first signs that they were actually working. Jack was on lithium, which worked fine once you found the proper dosage level, and continued treatment like a responsible adult, but Jack would feel better, figure that he no longer needed the encumbrance of taking a pill, then proceed to take his car apart piece by piece or try to plug an extension cord into a streetlight while yelling obscenities. My parents were constantly shuttling Jack between our house and the Veterans Administration hospital sixty miles south, where he would stay while he reacclimated to his medications, only to be picked up and brought home, where the cycle would begin again. Through thirteen-year-old eyes, I could see the toll it took on my parents, the strain it caused between them, and I, come hell or hotter hell, was determined that I was not going to add to their burden.

There was nothing altruistic in keeping my depression a secret. It wasn't stoic or admirable. It was simple problem avoidance, which always works out, right? I was deathly afraid that not only was I going to turn into Jack, but that I was evil to boot. My church experience had taught me that evil is bad and should be cast out, but it was inside me. Ergo, I should be cast out to wander aimlessly with just a staff and goat's bladder full of wine. Back then it was easier to hide my depression, because it wasn't a constant presence it moved in and out of my life like a bad case of crabs. Each time it would disappear I hoped that it was the last I'd ever have to experience it, but it would come back bigger and stronger and always last longer than the time before. Each emergence of my dark companion was followed by my asking God to intercede on my behalf, to end the suffering that I was experiencing, but relief never came. I know, believe me, I hear all the thumpers now: "God was only giving you what you could handle" or "During this time he was carrying you through the sand."

Here's the deal, the way I see it. If God is indeed the one who's handing out the challenges we are to overcome, then he is absolutely giving some more than they can handle. It's called suicide, and it's a real thing. I don't believe that God gave me depression, just like I don't believe he gave my mother cancer. I have never blamed him or shaken my fist while cursing him for making so many assholes. Needless to say, my relationship with God is complicated, and the church has done nothing but add further complexities to it. I have just never understood how an all-knowing, all-powerful entity would create such imperfect creatures, then require them to live their lives to seemingly impossible standards in order to have a relationship. I don't believe that God loves only Christians or people that only obey his every command. I think that is man's bullshit that he embellished the Word with to keep some people out of the country club pool. I think he loves everybody, no matter how their minds work, whom they love, or whom they pray to. Keep in mind that I am not or do I claim to be a theologian. Obviously, I will face judgment for my beliefs at some point just as you, and I'm good with that.

I understand that there are two sides to a coin and that my opinion is based on my own biases and experiences, but in my estimation, the glue that holds the modern church together is guilt. Upon reaching the age of majority I attended church out of guilt, took my wife and kids out of guilt, and paid tithes to the church out of guilt. I went on mission trips and wanted to be a church leader, working hard to be a "man of God" in large part due to guilt I felt for not living up to the example set for me by my parents. Don't get me wrong I believe in God and that truly righteous people exist and are good. I believe far, far less in the church or the provisional sanctimony it provides, or in the congregation members who raise their arms in praise, then their middle finger as they drive out the church parking lot.

If you are a depression sufferer that is comforted by prayer and religion, please, I beg of you, keep praying, don't stop attending services, and be involved and present in your spirituality. My experience should never sway anyone in their beliefs. If anything, I want to increase my spiritual exposure and would like to explore alternative paths to a relationship with God. I don't believe there is a God size hole in my heart, just saying that made me want to throw up in my mouth, but when my mind is stronger and has found calm and peace through time and meditation, then I will seek God out not because of guilt or to portray a societal image of piety but for a true, genuine relationship.

So this Sunday, like Sundays for years before, I will not be dressing up in my finest and taking my family to church. I've worked through the guilt, dealt with the fallout that comes with being an unrepentant backslider. I no longer feel the need to justify my actions like I once did, mostly because I found that I was just trying to give myself an excuse to not do something that has been indoctrinated in me to do. I discovered how, at least in this instance, to tell myself that it's okay to live my life by my beliefs and not the beliefs, wishes, or desires of someone else, no matter how high in regard I hold them. I have learned a couple things in my life. One is that seahorses are monogamous and will swim around cutely holding each other's tails. The other is that it is pure folly to never say never, so I may end up someday a member of a congregation again, especially if some control is achieved in this constant battle between my ears, but it won't be to serve an image of what a "Christian" man should be. It will be to enhance and build my relationship with God.

I'm not sure what is going to alienate me more from you, what I just said or what I am about to say. Between the months of August and February, there is another irritating occurrence that happens on Sundays that has been an irritant since I was just a lad, the National Football League. I know that there are people who live for professional football and the joy that can only be experienced by watching overpaid large sweaty men commit violence on each other while eating like a shredder with the Feds at the door. Don't get me wrong, I love college football. I love my home team and can be found supporting them by yelling at elevated levels through the television at the referees and sometimes the coaches. I enjoy the purity and unpredictability of college football. I can tell myself that these are student athletes working hard for their future and that it's not about money, although I clearly know that it is, but I like the illusion; it doesn't make me feel as slimy.

The local college team plays in a stadium that is less than three miles from my house, the nearest professional stadium is over three hundred miles away in a different state, and when I was in my developmental stage as an NFL viewer, that team sucked, so I never acquired a positive affiliation that I could carry with me. Many boring rainy Sunday afternoons were spent around a TV set watching teams I didn't care about, just wishing they would just finish the stupid game so I could watch *The Muppet Show*. As I grew older, I became more and more indifferent to the NFL. Sure, I'll watch some games, especially around playoff time, and the Super Bowl for me is way more about the commercials and way less about the actual game, which often is overrated AF. If there is any licensed NFL merch in my house, it was given as a gift and I haven't donated it yet to charity. Don't get me wrong, I'm not taking a stand against the NFL, not trying to offer any commentary designed to sway opinions for or against. I just don't know what the big deal is. I've wanted to be a part of the hype and excitement. I want to act like it's fourth-grade lunch hour, and I can heat and play with my friends, but that has always eluded me.

Therein lies the rub. I have realized in writing this that my problem with Sunday in general has always been a feeling of disenfranchisement. I have witnessed people receiving an enormous amount of joy and satisfaction from activities that have left me wanting. I feel I'm outside, alone and cold, creepily watching happy, better-dressed people smiling and laughing and cutting roast beast. That may be a little dark. Try this: it's like arriving at Disney World after counting down the days for months and feeling the jubilation as you see Mickey Mouse, then as you go to give him a hug, he kicks you square in the nuts with those big fucking shoes. The joy that people feel on Sunday, the peace, the redemption, and comfort, has always evaded me, and that has not gone unnoticed by my depression, as coincidentally my melancholy increases significantly.

Like I have always said and will always say, depression is diabolical and will use every ounce of leverage it can bring against you. It had a field day with the whole church guilt thing, almost getting its way on one occasion. It will use the "missing out" angle on occasion, but even my depression seems to give few shits about the NFL. The point being that if something bothers you it can and will be used against you, and the only thing that will stop it is coming to a resolution. Not the resolution in the New Year's "not going to touch my nethers ever again" sense, but in the "I need to come to a resolution about guilt I feel when no guilt feeling is required" kind of thing. Keep in mind that I'm a guilt freak. I horde the stuff like it's edible, so it was incredibly hard and took a lot of self-discipline and positive talk to move beyond this particular guilt, but once I did, it deprived my depression of that weapon and rendered it ineffective. Now if I can just do that to the six hundred seventy-eight other guilt issues patiently waiting their turn.

MONDAY, JUNE 29, 2020

I don't think we need to talk about what five in the morning on a Monday feels like, do I? I think I made some of my feelings clear yesterday when I was going off. I hope that wasn't too much. I was afraid I was going to lose you. Do you know who absolutely loves Monday mornings? That's right, the three furballs of the apocalypse. Having not had a walk since Friday, the Dog Walkers Union Local 819 allows me to take the weekends off. They are out of their damn minds with anticipation and shoot through the door like the opening gun for the Iditarod just sounded. As we round the first corner, Hondo is literally choking himself to death. We all make it home safely, due in large part to my superior mushing skills, but I have only one thing on my mind, coffee.

Oh, how I rejoice in the simple elegance and wonder that is my first cup of coffee on a Monday morning. It makes my head sing and my heart flutter. It is my reason, my purpose, and my porpoise; coffee is my porpoise. Did that just get weird? Sorry. I'm going over the plan for the day and all in all it's a low-key Monday. I have some items requiring a check mark in a box. Talking with Nancy about Bill's condition is definitely on the list, along with some Zooms and emails. Of course, I will also follow the prime directive, which in this sense means spending some time on me, doing some meditation and contemplation, and getting my shirt wet.

Yesterday during meditation, the Calm lady with the amazing voice talked about how our minds can be like small unruly children needing to be herded and controlled during our time of mindfulness. I was like, "Sister, please, you're milking the bull here," but through

54

her teaching, I began to understand that control is possible, you can rein in hyperactive thoughts, and that it's not as hard as I thought it would be. I learned that meditation is an active endeavor. It requires attention and focus but to various degrees of intensity. Just sitting calmly with your hands cupped in your lap makes you enlightened like eating a plate of wood makes you a beaver. It truly takes effort to make it look effortless. I find myself surprisingly into this mindfulness thing. I believe that it holds tremendous promise as an arrow in the quiver in my depression fight. It's still new to me. I'm like a novice's personal assistant, but it feels positive, and I like positive.

I've always taken a hands-on approach to my depression, especially since I came just five-inch pounds of force from propelling a small metal projectile through my brain stem. If you're waiting for our suicide talk, it's coming. I just need to be ready to talk about that topic, and today's not that day. That being said, side B of that suicide record is about not killing yourself; it's about being proactive about your survival and taking control of depression management.

Okay, what in the name of Seymour Dix is depression management, you ask? Great question, thank you for asking it, because it gives me the opportunity to talk about depression management. Aside from sounding like a course you can take from International Correspondence Schools, depression management is developing tools to help you in your fight and creating awareness of when to use them. I will tell you of my experience, but I highly recommend that you come up with your own system that is specific to you and your unique experience. I have developed for myself a rabbit hole scale (RHS), a vertical scale that starts out wide at its mouth and narrows the lower down it goes, much like an inverted pyramid scheme. Being above ground is preferred, both on my scale and in real life. This level requires nothing out of the ordinary besides maintenance and monitoring, making sure to exercise and meditate and drink coffee.

The first narrowing level within the hole on my scale I named optimistically "just dropping by." This level is characterized as a situation or event that occurs darkening our spirit or outlook. My experience has shown that for good or bad, this is a very temporary level. From here with diligence I will be able to pump the bilges by taking a walk or working a puzzle, perhaps painting a picture. This is a crucial point and should exemplify the need for constant vigilance because depression is like the *Titanic*—it's long, kills people, and is hard to steer. Turning your depression, if it's anything like mine, will take a bit of work and patience, but the early effort will be worth it. If you ignore the early signs of trouble you, do so at your peril, because as I said, "just dropping by" is a transitory level. You will either hit the up arrow or find yourself on the next level down before you know it.

That next level on the RHS is called the moody blues. This level is not named in honor of the band. As a matter of fact, the song "Knights in White Satin" makes me want to find someone with feathered hair and punch them in the face. No, this level is basically named in honor of the way I'm usually feeling when I'm at this level. I have been here many times, and it's akin to a wet fart. You're pretty sure you didn't shit your pants, but you should probably take care of business. Panic is not required here, but effort is. A walk is not going to get it done, this level requires a coordinated attack of multiple activities coupled with talking. A bigger project, whether that's art, or construction, or writing, is just what the "not a medical professional" ordered. Just be careful *not* to attempt something you haven't done before or that may carry a high degree of failure because that would be what we in the nonmedical profession call "bad."

I cannot say this enough. Early and continued effort will be rewarded, but be patient. Remember that your depression may have itty-bitty rudders for as large as it is, so it may happen so slow that you don't feel yourself getting better, but stick with it. The alternative is to give up and sink even deeper down the rabbit hole to a level appropriately called the third level of hell. This is a nod to every depressive's favorite thirteenth-century Italian poet Dante Alighieri, who created the seven circles of hell, based on the seven deadly sins, which doesn't really jive with what I what I was after since the third circle is about gluttony, unless you attempt to eat yourself happy, which I have, unsuccessfully.

If you find yourself on this level, plan on checking in, it's going to take a while to climb out. It is on this level that I first realized that I could not dig myself out of a hole. I would not come out in China where a family with no children would take me, name me Yuehan-shimisi, and allow me to start fresh. This level is no joke, and panic is definitely in order as you are far closer to the abyss that to being above ground. A firm slap across the face followed by a regimented routine of talking to a professional, exercise, mental activities, talking to nonprofessionals, and singing show tunes is required. You have to be absolutely committed at this point. You should be taking time off work, gathering your support around you, doing what doctors tell you to do, and genuinely working to get better. Keep in mind that any asshole can be miserable and die alone. It takes character and courage to ask for help and humility to accept it.

The last level on the tour today is truly the vilest and should be avoided at all costs, and I do mean that literally—do everything within your power and ability to never set foot here. I have been here twice and both times was fortunate to make it out alive. This level is called proper fucked, and if you're here, you are. Once in this realm, all bets are off, and everything is in play. The longer you stay here, the closer you get to being dead, and I mean that in all seriousness. This is walking a minefield blindfolded or playing Russian roulette with a machine gun. You have to get the fuck out immediately. Call the National Suicide Prevention Lifeline at 1-800-273-8255 right fucking now. Call your best friend and tell them to take you to the emergency room. You cannot get out of this level alone or on your terms. You need immediate, significant help, and you need it right now. If you think this level wants to eat your soul while you watch through horrified eyes, then you get an idea of the evil that lives here. This is the death zone. Every hour you spend here increases you chances of killing yourself. The longer your exposure, the more desperate you become, until at some point you don't care about anything else.

If you've ever gone through a personal safety course or have been involved in self-defense, chances are you've been trained in threat awareness and assessment and conflict avoidance. When you walk into a room, you find the exits, know your pinch points, and run a scenario in your head. You need to do the same thing with your depression, have a real time awareness of where on your scale you are, and know what your triggers are and what tools work for you. There is unquestionably no substitute for proactivity, but it will not prevent episodes or effects of depression. Your darkness isn't just going to give up and go away just because you're ready, ever. That bastard will just wait and watch, knowing at some point your guard will lower. Nobody can stand watch twenty-four/seven, which is why depression management is so crucial.

Then Lisa's phone rings. Talk about apropos to the topic of the day. Lisa just got off the phone with Nancy and Bill is now at home but on hospice. While I see this as a win as far as control and closure for family and friends in the time of COVID-19, it is an acceptance of the inevitability of what is to come, and that hurts. I understand death, I have fixated on my own and have experienced it with people I love, and I realize that it's as much a part of life as sunshine and oxygen. I am also aware that it can bring peace and closure just as it does anguish and longing. I grieve more for the death of the fight, the dying of that magical internal spark that makes Bill or any of us who we are. While the body will pass in its own time, once that spark is gone, once the eyes close for the last time, all that remains on this earth of that person is what fuel they left for others to feed their own sparks. My heart aches already for the void Bill will leave, but he has fed my spark more than he will ever know, so for that I am grateful.

We make plans to make the drive south on Sunday. It may be the last time we see him on this side of the veil, but we won't act like it. We will sit and talk and laugh and once more be blessed by Bill's easy smile and positive attitude. I'm sure at some point, when it's time to say goodbye, that tears will flow, that hugs will last longer, that emotions will overcome. I know that my depression, like the insensitive cocksucker that it is, will be there in that moment too, like a vulture waiting for me to weaken, waiting for me to level down. I will need to be vigilant and on my game, constantly assessing where I am on my scale and in my head. At the end of the day, that is all I can do, that and find someone with feathered hair, just in case.

Good morning. It's good to see you, hope you are well rested. Me? I've been sleeping like a delicious houseguest at Jeff Dahmer's house. I've been spending more and more time dredging the soil where I buried my issues. Every night at the stroke of "I have to pee," the ghosts of depression past drop by for a chat. Sometimes I have vivid historical reenactments of things that have happened in sepia-colored dreams, sometimes the notions just pop into my brain as I lay my head back on the pillow. Mind you, I take every precaution. I shuffle my feet like I'm shackled, so I don't step on anything or stub my toes. I keep my eyes closed as much as possible and don't turn on the light, hoping more than relying that the payload will hit its target. Still, like an impatient kid on Christmas morn, waiting for the earliest indications of dawn. My issues are like "Hey, bro, you up? I need to talk." I never get up, never look at my phone. I just lie there thinking about the best way to not think, suffering in silence. Of course, I fall fast asleep when Lisa starts to stir and then twenty minutes later feel like I will kill anyone who tries to get me out of this bed by pressing my thumbs grossly into their eye sockets, but then, my mantra, and I get my ass up. "Once more into the fray."

I wish that they made a pill that could give me the same feeling as my first morning cup of coffee, the welcoming feeling that the hot mug warms my hands as I bring it to my lips for that first tentative sip. The rich aroma of a perfectly roasted bean wafts through my nostrils, making my little brain gnomes sing and dance. Now I've been around. I know that there are pills that offer euphoric properties, but they are far too costly, and I'm not talking just money. My wisdom teeth weren't removed from my head until I was in my late thirties.

By then they had attached themselves to my jaw so securely that the only way to remove them was by holding my head at an eighteen-degree angle while a Lipizzaner stallion kicked me in the face. The pain was significant, and for that I was prescribed a week of hydrocodone. This was the good shit, the shit you could sell on the street, the shit that not only kills the pain but the all of the pains family just to send a message to other pain.

If a pharmaceutical aimed at depression worked as well as the opioid painkillers, we'd be discussing the topic of whether or not cereal is in fact really just cold soup and not depression at all. The problem is that at their most efficacious, depression meds can be a very sticky wicket. What we need to agree upon at this moment that by having a discussion about depression medications that we are heading down a path that is fraught with hazard. It needs to be understood that what I'm about to say is based on my own understanding and experience in my life. I have no medical or pharmaceutical training or education. I'm not even wearing underwear, so before making changes to any treatment plan you may be considering, first consult your professional and be honest with them and open to suggestion. I say this not out of concern for the covering of my ass but out of my own experience. Adding or changing medications or dosages can have a serious impact on your mental well-being and should in consultation with professional help and an abundance of caution. Believe me, I have personally witnessed and starred in shit-shows produced and directed by changing meds and dosages willy-nilly.

As of the moment that I write these words, I am not taking any antidepressants, and there is a very good reason why. Have you ever watched an advertisement for a depression medication on the TV? I can't see how you could've missed any, since there's at least one every time they go to break, unless you have one of those fast-forward thingamajiggers. After they show the sad person missing out on life, taking the pills, then smiling again miraculously, they go into side effects, which always include death and of course diarrhea. The problem for the drug company is that during the drug trials, there will be at least one poor soul who commits suicide, which isn't a side effect; it's a fucking tragedy.

Unfortunately, I'm firmly in the percentage of people who experience suicidal thoughts, ideations, or actions when under the effects of medication. I'm sure for some it's because of their unique brain chemistry. For me, I think it's because of something else. I had to learn to deal with depression from an early age, and since it was my "secret," I had to develop ways to combat it without relying on outside help, and that is what I did. When the truth about my darkness made its way to daylight, and I truly sought professional guidance, I was put on various medications of differing dosages, each one making it harder and harder to fight my depression in the manner that I had become accustomed to. As a result of this, I would keep dangerously leveling down the rabbit hole, creeping closer and closer to the abyss. I had to come off each one in order to regain my ability to effectively fight back.

Here's the problem as I see it. Depression may be a result of a chemical imbalance in the head. I know that this has definitely been a prevailing theory since my early days, but there is so much more that factor in, like lifestyle, sleep, digestion, and stress levels, that make immediate effectiveness unlikely. I remember reading at one point that only 25 percent of patients reported feeling better upon starting a pharmaceutical treatment. Keep in mind that my source for all the information I pass along as my own originates directly from the internetz, the z is just to look cool to hipsters. If it was solely a chemical imbalance, say serotonin levels were low or out of balance, it stands to reason that adding a selective serotonin reuptake inhibitor would stabilize that imbalance and solve the problem, then why, according to my shoddy research, would it only work on a quarter of the people who are prescribed to? Obviously to my untrained brain, there is other stuff that is also playing a role. Now this is like saying Moses parted the Red Sea because he never learned to swim as a child and had left his water wings back in Egypt. While there may be a debatable element of truth to that, there are too many factors at play to make a conclusion without further understanding.

I say this more for you, the person who is struggling, who may be thinking about talking with your healthcare provider about how you feel, who may be questioning adding a medication to your treatment plan. The first thing that I would say is good for you, talk away, and tell them all your thoughts and feelings. If they want to look toward prescribing medications, go for it, but do so with these things in mind. That little pill with the long made-up name may not work for you, especially immediately. Don't expect to take the pill and close your eyes, and suddenly your life is filled with magic dolphin-riding monkeys. Depression pharmacology is a long game, so take your pills every day and settle in, unless that is, if it starts to make your mindset far worse or you begin to feel yourself losing control. If that happens, stop everything, stop playing Pokémon, stop making ramen noodles, stop foraging for nuts, and call your doctor. Don't stop taking the meds unless you're told to do so by a person with letters after their name, because sometimes it can actually make it worse.

And for the love of Grandma's warm strawberry rhubarb pie, or whatever it is that you hold holy, under no circumstances, if the routine you are on is working, assume that you are cured and therefore no longer require being under care. That is a complete dickhead move and is a slap in the face of all of us who will never experience that singular joy. Just understand that there is no cure for depression, just treatments, so if you feel relief in what you are doing, then don't stop, ever. If you haven't yet found relief, don't stop trying, keep an open dialogue with your healthcare provider, try adding an antipsychotic in tandem with your treatment, or talk about increasing a dosage. Also, understand that there are amazing activities that you can do without a prescription, such as breathe, meditate, exercise, walk on a beach, let a puppy bite you with those sharp little piranha teeth, lay in the sun, tell someone you love them, let them love you back, drink a goddamn cup of coffee, and just live.

I don't care how old you are. If you live with depression, you're an adult. If you're younger than eighteen, I'm sorry for saying "fuck" so much, but mostly I'm sorry because your childhood is, for all intents and purposes, over. You are going to have to deal with adult things and adult feelings, and you're going to have to behave like an adult. Adults need to be responsible for their actions, need to understand that what happens in their lives, good or bad, requires their implicit permission. As much as we want to feel sorry for ourselves from time to time, it's not a treatment option and does much more harm than good. For whatever reason, either fate or cosmic kismet, you have been selected to carry a burden, and with that burden comes the choice to become that burden, be defined by that burden, or rise despite of your burden. Electing to rise is the noblest of choices but by far the most demanding and challenging. Rising will not happen alone or in a vacuum. It will take all the tools you can muster and building a support structure of family, friends, professionals, and at least one amazing baker, you know, for the biscuits and pies.

Once you reach equilibrium with your treatment and depression, know that the fight isn't over, far from it. Tactics will have to be revised, dosages changed, maybe starting yoga, or finishing the ice cream. Be ready and able to adapt to what that literal sly devil has in store. I myself have tried multiple attempts at different medications, one just a couple of years ago. A setback occurred, as they do, and I was open to giving a combination of medications a go. The attempt was a failure requiring the immediate suspension of the meds, but the shot was taken, and I would rather try, fail, and know than deprive myself an option.

Holy jumping up and down Martha! Enough of the meds already, I know sometimes I get lecturey about stuff, and I sound like I'm giving a PowerPoint presentation to tourists on a time-share junket who really just want to go to the pool. Don't get me wrong, today has been something of a washout, having my two Zoom meetings that both have to be rescheduled, but sometimes you're the ass, and sometimes you're the saddle. I did get something done. I got to go into the wellness center and get a plantar wart frozen off my foot. Let me tell you something—depression is a donkey sucker, but the constant, sustained, irritating pain from a plantar wart makes you want to chew your own foot off. Why do you think that so many pirates had peg legs? I'll tell you, damp environments with boots made of unbreathing leather and socks made of seaweed or woven human hair. It's no wonder they would dangle their warty feet in shark-infested waters.

I was actually really looking forward to this appointment, working out has been more painful and less gainful as of late. My biggest concern about the whole process is my odor insecurities. I've probably not spoken of this particular issue, and I know this may sound strange, but I would rather not have anyone smell me, unless I don't smell bad. I'm not sure when or where I picked up this particular issue but I'm a sweater. If I was a sideshow attraction, I would be the human sprinkler. I would run on a treadmill, then shake like a dog, spraying the audience with droplets of sweat while they ooh and aah. As cool as I'm sure you think this is, sweat and body odor want to run through a field of daisy's holding hands. You must deny them the opportunity. So shortly before my appointment, I wash my feet, apply some of Lisa's fancy lotion that smells like driving a lavender bush through a car wash, put on clean dry socks, and head for the door.

In this time of "serious" medical issues the staff seemed relieved to be dealing with something so mundane, but they took all precautions and got an accurate picture of my overall health before having me take off my shoes and socks and sit on the exam table. They use liquid nitrogen to freeze the wart off, but first, she explained that she would have to remove some dead skin around it, or it wouldn't kill it properly, then promptly took out the sharpest-looking instrument I had ever seen, like something you would use to threaten a knife. She told me, "I'm going to trim the skin back. Let me know if you feel any pain."

To which I thought, "Holy shit, she's going to cut my foot with that thing and I'm going to feel it. I don't want to feel it. What do I say when I feel it? Ouch? Aargh?"

By the time I had figured I would just say "Owwie" but in a deeper voice, she was done with the whole procedure. She put a simple dressing on the exposed wound and headed out the door. I put my sock and shoe back on and followed suit.

Today was a "meh" day. If it wasn't for killing a wart, I feel I wouldn't have accomplished much other than a discussion about depression meds, which was good, don't get me wrong, but it wasn't what I had hoped it would be, and that's okay. If we ate warm strawberry rhubarb pie every day, it wouldn't be special.

WEDNESDAY, JULY 1, 2020

I'm a blessed man leading a blessed life. I feel very fortunate to have made it to midlife without first dying. So many days younger me wanted to end it, make it stop by my own hand or through alcohol. I would have missed so much, spending time with those I love, building a business, traveling, helping others where I can. So much would have been lost and wasted. I stand before you, a man honestly saying that I have no major regrets in my life. I'm not haunted by things I've done or opportunities I didn't take, mostly due to the fact that I am still alive.

Now, minor regrets, I got those. I don't really think it's possible to go through life without any regrets whatsoever. I mean, even Gandhi wished he had better shoes. I regret my mom getting rid of my original *Star Wars* action figures and my comic books. I regret buying the parachute pants and not buying the brisket, every time. There are too many to count, but I would say my biggest small regret is not taking the fullest advantage of summer while it's here. Normal years I work straight through the week. We get Big Man J on Saturdays for a visit. That leaves Sunday to enjoy all summer has to offer while catching up on the house chores, finishing laundry, preparing for Monday, et cetera. Before I can put out an announcement looking for my missing tan, storm clouds are moving in from the west, bringing with it the fall chill in the air. This year I told Lisa that I'm going to take a day off during the week so we can do some fun summer stuff that our area has to offer. I mean, it's not like we're going anywhere, and the highlight of yesterday was getting a wart removed.

Oregon in summer is an absolute outdoor sportsman's paradise in the summer. I know that Louisiana claims to be the Sportsman's Paradise, boldly announcing it on their license plates, but I've been there in the summer, and with that humidity, the sport better be at night or in the shower. Sometimes the biggest problem is choosing from all of the likely options. Lisa's friend Storm was talking about going golfing, so we decided on a trip up the McKenzie River to a golf course with amazing views, figuring we haven't golfed in years, so may as well get some amazing views while trying to find erroneously struck golf balls. After that we'd head east a few miles and take a hike to the famous Blue Pool. It was set, summer wasn't going to pass us by this year, and it felt good, until I saw how many spiders were living in my golf bag.

I fought the urge to light the bag on fire, which is my go-to for dealing with spiders, and started cleaning. I felt like an archeologist there was so much dust. It seems Tutankhamen preferred a lob wedge to a pitching wedge, interesting. When Noah heard about the outing, he wanted to go, giving us a fourth, which was nice because they wouldn't throw some random asshole with us when we checked in, and I've always been paired with assholes, never just regular holes. So we were set, two people who haven't golfed in years; Storm, who has done some golfing but still not enough to understand you don't use a driver for every shot; and Noah, who, having competed in Special Olympics golf skills events in pre-pandemic years, is probably our ringer. Our foursome is every pro shop's worst nightmare, a real hole clogger, and we're planning to walk the course.

We decide on the drive up to just play nine holes since we will be hiking later in the day, then make the one mistake rusty golfers should never make. We arrive at the course only ten minutes before tee time, barely giving the ladies time to change clothes to coordinate outfits, let alone hitting a bucket or practicing a few putts. My first warm-up golf swing in over seven hundred days was after I'd teed up my ball on hole number one. Two foursomes were already lined up sitting in their carts behind us, just waiting to run us down the moment our pace slowed. Those who know me understand that I don't normally mind the spotlight shining down on me, I can handle it, but the first tee, when you're the first away, and all eyes are on you makes your anus pucker a little.

I took an extra swing or two, then lined up, took the club back, and let muscle memory take the wheel. Amazingly I hit the ball flush, and it flew well past the women's tee, which was my primary goal, being in mixed company, wink. Storm and Lisa were looking at me clapping. I gave them a nod like there was never any doubt. It turns out I was the long driver of the group with Storm, Lisa, and Noah all mishitting their tee shots and ending up on the course somewhere between "Damn" and "Shit." There is an unwritten rule in golf. Well, there's actually a shitload of unwritten rules in golf. Google "Texas rule" and ask yourself if this would actually get you watching golf on TV. The one I'm talking about, however, is "If you're gonna suck, suck fast!" That is exactly what we did, moving purposefully and keeping a decent pace, especially since everyone else on the course was in a cart.

Golf is not a sport; it's a skills competition. I know there are people who will argue this point, but there is no inherent athleticism required other than walking between skill challenges and wearing wide belts. In my younger days, you had to be infirm or have polio to ride in a cart. "Dead man riding" we wouldn't say because *The Green Mile* hadn't come out yet, but it would've been funny in a callous way. The whole benefit to golf was in the walk. If you don't walk, you might as well be bowling, another nonsport skills competition. I firmly believe that the Disney movie *Wall-E*, though not one of my favorites, accurately predicts where our society is heading, and it is playing out before my very eyes. Sloppy humans letting machines carry them so they can drink and eat more and do less are all around us. Wake up, people; the fucking machines are not your friends, unless it's a coffee maker.

We moved from shot to shot, playing "ready golf," enjoying the day. Every so often I would hit the ball just like old times, and it felt good. Of the four of us, I have the most golf experience, but that came to an end in 2008. At one point, like every other tucked-in-shirt-, one-glove-wearing asshole, I thought I could go somewhere with golf. I would hang out at golf courses, check out the newest clubs and merchandise, hit buckets before hitting buckets, and chip and putt, pretending each shot was for the win. The problem was that the more I practiced, the better I became. The better I became, the more pressure I put on myself. The more pressure I put on myself, the worse I played. The worse I played, the more depressed I became.

Golf actually contributed heavily to one of my worst and fastest downward spirals. It was a rough patch personally, and financially and holding up a big check with a bigger smile was what I wanted. I mean, I'd broke eighty a few times, so how much harder could it be? I immersed myself in the attempt with a singular vision, forsaking most other aspects of my life, including my depression. I was so sure that the activity was "good" for me and was keeping the darkness at bay, when in actuality I blinded myself to its advances, and before I knew it, I was "average" as a golfer and under siege as a human. I tell you this as a cautionary tale of dreaming and large check envy. Don't let a fixation, even a seemingly healthy one, leave the back door unlocked and castle unguarded. By the time I crawled out of the hole, I was stronger and wiser and had given up on my dream of wearing an ugly blazer and holding a trophy while people clapped for me. When my dad died in 2008, I lost my father, my friend, my mentor in business and in life, and my constant golf buddy. Since his passing, I could count the number of times I've golfed on my fingers and toes and still have digits left to spare, in case I ever need to show my fealty to a mob boss or something.

I took it upon myself to keep our group on task and pace and lead us from hole to hole, cognizant of the future citizens of the Spaceship Axiom lining up behind us. None of us kept score other than smiles beat frowns by a landslide, especially when the sun broke free from the tight hug of the clouds and the rays hit our faces. I hit a 148-yard approach with an eight iron within six feet of the flag on the sixth hole and putted in for par. A twinge of excitement and wonder crossed my mind: "What if." Thankfully, my following tee shot was so bad, it will only be found by future archeologists wondering what kind of egg they just found, reminding me to just be in the moment and have fun.

We finished the nine holes in just under two hours, which gave me a sense of accomplishment, way more for my herding abilities than for my golf prowess. If written on paper, our combined score would have been visible from space, but each of us hit some surprisingly amazing shots, which we happily recounted as we sat on the patio and ate our lunch. Talking about shared experiences is something humans love to do and, I feel, one of the most important things that depression takes from us. It's hard to share experience if you're on the couch with the shades drawn, and it's even harder to talk about it. I have tried on a couple of occasions to start a group where sufferers could get together, do art activities, and talk about what we had done, but the grip of depression is mighty strong, and nothing lasted. So if you know someone who suffers, get them out, and ask them to join in activity. If you are a sufferer and someone asked you to join them, say yes. Your depression won't like you going out, won't like you being around others, will hate if you talk, despise if it's about feelings, but that's the damn point.

About twenty miles up the road is the trailhead to the famous Blue Pool. I'm guessing it's famous because of the amazing riverside hike leading to the spectacular pool, but for all I know, it could be where Lewis caught Clark and Sacagawea skinny-dipping. I have been on this hike several times, but as is the theme of the day, it's been awhile. Even with the COVID-19 making its rounds throughout the world, the license plates lining the dirt road leading to the trailhead were from all over the country and Canada. The "road trip" was definitely enjoying a comeback, bringing back memories of twelve-hour days, hot uncomfortable cars, sleeping on pads, tacky tourist crap, and some of the best memories ever.

The two-mile hike to the pool, which is formed by an underwater river, is one of the most beautiful I've ever taken. It follows the river flowing out of the pool through an old growth forest and ancient lava flows from the prehistoric era of our state. It is a heavily traveled out and back trail, meaning you have two-way people and or mountain bike traffic to contend with as you walk the narrow path. One particular point of the trail, alongside river rapids, leads my brain to thoughts of my mom. One of the last things she told me before she died was that she wanted me to sit by a river. She loved sitting by a river or walking along the ocean. It was her happy place, where she could calm herself and talk with her Lord. She wanted me to experience the calming grace that she felt. One day I will honor her wishes, find a nice place to sit next to moving water, and just be. I don't know what I will do when this time comes. I guess just sit there until the spirit moves me to do something else, for some reason I'm in no hurry to fulfill this promise, and that is unlike me, so I know that there are other forces at play, so I push on.

Noah and I lead the way, pushing through the twisting roots and cragged lava flows, giving the ladies time to chat, which they did unceasingly. Topics ran the gamut from spray tans, to theoretical astrophysics, then back to how cute that skort looks. About fifty minutes after our shoes hit the path, we rounded a corner, gained elevation over uneven ground strewn with more elevated roots and boulders, and caught our first glimpse of the pool, and like always it didn't disappoint as the vivid topaz water glistened in the sunlight. Every time I see it, I'm reminded of Nehi Blue Cream Soda, one of my favorites growing up, that you can't get anymore because it was made of blue opium poppies or something. From where you first glimpse the pool it is a fifty- to sixty-foot drop to the crystal-clear water below. The pool itself is over thirty feet deep but you can see every detail of the bottom clearly. Many people over the years have jumped from above into the frigid water below, a few have died or had to be rescued because of injuries suffered in the attempt. If you are so inclined and want to jump in, there is a trail that leads to water's edge on the backside of the pool. Given the path is technical with trees and scree to traverse, and that Noah isn't the most sure-footed, and that the pool itself is just over thirty-eight degrees in temperature, we decide to wait to jump in until we're actually on fire.

The walk back always seems shorter to me for some reason, even though we covered the distance in the almost exact same time. Lisa prefers to drive and has done all of the driving today. She tells me it's nothing personal. She just likes being in control. I don't take it personally, which makes me wonder if I should, but then I go back to not taking it personally, especially since she is an amazing driver, and honestly, I'm only a defensive driver, if being a good offensive driver counts. We usually agree that if we need to arrive safely, Lisa will drive, and if we are fleeing a crime scene and need to get to the safe house fast, I'm behind the wheel. So I sit in the back with Noah to again to allow the ladies greater conversation dynamics as we head home.

Today was a huge success, we accomplished quite a bit by not accomplishing anything. We enjoyed our time together and created more memories that a normal working Wednesday. I want you to know something, that dealing with depression no matter how often or severe is not a penal punishment; you are not serving a sentence for wrongdoing, so many people think that smiles, fun, and depression are mutually exclusive, but that is a choice to be made by each sufferer. Balance is important, and if you are a depression sufferer, you will see darkness, and you will feel sadness and anxiety. It comes naturally with the membership card and decoder ring. It's up to you to balance the scales, to seek peace, light, and happiness. Make the most of every opportunity that presents itself to do just that. Today was a shot of B_{12} and ground rhino horn right to the veins, and I loved every minute of it.

Thursday, July 2, 2020

Have you ever slept in when you weren't planning on it? This morning I woke up with a jolt. I knew something was off. I reached for my phone, knocking over the lamp for the hundredth time, righted it with a curse, and then tapped my screen and was shocked to see 5:45 a.m. displayed in bright, bold numbers. I sat up like a squirrel was biting my nipples, thinking "Holy shit! The day's half over." I jumped out of bed and scrambled to the bathroom. In full make-up-time mode, I put some pressure behind my flow, making the tip of my penis burn a little, then try to calm myself as I throw some clothes on and make the bed. I don't know why I get so worked up when this happens. I don't set an alarm or have to punch an early clock. I could literally sleep another hour and a half and no other human being would give a single shit. But still, here I am disheveled, sleep in my eyes and a stingy penis trying to catch up.

You know who cares about my wake-up time? The three dwarf dingoes waiting for their tour of the outback, which makes me nervous because the later we leave, the greater chance we'll run into other likeminded people and their furry bosses, and no one wants that to happen more than me. The way that these three canine thugs act when they realize that there are other dogs living within barking distance is embarrassing at best. At worst I expect a bill for doggy therapy sessions with Cesar Milan. In my mind it plays out like this, we're walking down the street, when suddenly walking toward us on the opposite side, a dog and its employee. They pull harder as the distance closes as if drawn by a magnetic force toward destiny or humping. In unison and in human voices turned to eleven they say,

"Hey! You're a dog! We're all dogs! What's your name! Whoa, what's that smell? Is that your butthole? Do you mind? Wait, where are you going? When can we see you again?" The other dog walks by without saying anything, kinda elegant and knows it, probably French. A single tear rolls down the nose of the three small dogs simultaneously; as they drop, they merge into one normal size tear, which lands softly on the ground where now a single crimson rose grows. What? I need coffee.

It was a rocky start, I'm not going to lie, but this Rainforest Blend from South America with its rich smoky aroma and smooth mouthfeel is righting a listing ship. When I was in basic training, I had nightmares about sleeping through reveille, or mustering naked, like either of those would actually happen, but maybe that is the genesis of my oversleeping issue. The brain is a fickle little imp sometimes. I will meditate later on the mental importance that I place on certain aspects of my life, and honestly, I feel like a grown-up, when I say things like I will meditate later. Of any day this week, today would have been best to sleep in anyway I have no meetings until later and no issues waiting for my input, hell I could go back to bed right now, but then I realize that no, I actually couldn't. I have placed so much importance on getting up and getting moving, not giving my depression an easy foothold, like mornings, that I'm like ugly wallpaper. Once I'm up, you're stuck.

I'm also like a lifelong subscriber, I have issues. How do you feel about phone calls? No, what I mean is how does the phone ringing make you feel? I get a twinge of nervousness almost every time my phone rings, or in actuality, vibrates since I never have the ringer on, because of my interruption issues. If I'm in the middle of a workout class and my phone rings, of course I don't answer because I'm not a douchebag, but what I will do is obsess about it unceasingly until I am able to get to my phone. I'm on the rower, thinking that someone's got a gun to the caller's head and their only hope of survival is me picking up my phone, or someone's on *Who Wants to be a Millionaire* and I'm their "phone a friend" lifeline, and I'm uncaringly doing sweaty hammer curls listening to Britney Spears. I've had some serious calls in my life, don't get me wrong, but I've never had a life-or-death situation, yet every fucking time the phone lights up, I fixate on a clock ticking down on a bomb while I selfishly sweat droplets of shame. I realize that so much of my existence is spent trying to not disappoint people, and my depression is all over that shit, exploiting and exaggerating to the point a grown man is afraid of his phone. Wow, I just worked that out, which is both awesome and pathetic. The question is what am I going to do about it? The answer is, I don't know. You can't just stop a train loaded with shit, a shit train. You have to slow it down first, so I will have to devise an ill-conceived, complicated plan, if that's okay with you?

God, this thinking thing sucks. Now I'm reflecting on how I will often leave an event early, even if I'm having fun, just so I can beat the traffic. I won't even stay for the "grand finale" of the fireworks show, preferring to imagine them violently blowing up the sky on my way to the car. I'm writing this slowly in hopes that the answer why will magically pop into my mind upon reflection, but like Yukon Cornelius said upon licking his pickaxe, "nothing." I know I don't like being stuck in a crowd, and I hate traffic, so maybe it's just that easy, but it just doesn't feel right. There has got to be a deeper explanation. Most issues I've been finding out revolve around control or disappointing people, which leads me to believe that the real culprit in this case is global freaking warming. Just kidding, global warming doesn't exist; it's just a left-wing propaganda tool to distract from the real culprit, government mind-control microchips injected in vaccines. Just kidding, more. This has all the markings of a classic control issue. By leaving early, I am exerting control over the variables of traffic and crowding. Plus I think there is a smaller element that by believes I am winning if I beat everyone else home.

Of course, when you suffer from depression and you spend any time actively thinking, you thoughts inevitably will fall upon your darkness. It seems to be a life of climbing, reaching one false summit after the next, achieving new heights but never quite reaching an apex. The trick is to not be consumed by the climb ahead but to enjoy the view you have achieved, because even a false summit allows you to enjoy the beauty around you. I have never wanted to be that dark, negative guy that brings the gloom to every room, which should be an Eminem lyric. Many people have no idea of the struggles that I endure behind a smiling face and positive attitude. A false face is something that every functioning depressive has fashioned for themselves to wear whenever they leave home. We don't wear a mask as an front or a deception but out of an absolute desire to achieve a degree of normalcy in our lives, but end up feeling like Cinderella, waiting for the stroke of midnight when we'll be seen for what we really are, dark and different.

Here's the deal, though. I love positivity and am a firm believer in the power of positive thought and actions. I would assume that a lot of depressed people feel the same, considering that if I'm anything, I'm average and being so I would represent a large piece of the sad pie chart. I value optimism and the constructive nature of an affirmative mindset versus the draining, eroding effects of pessimism, in its simplest form is making lemonade instead of throwing lemons at cars from an overpass.

When you think about it, finding clinically depressed people who believe in the power of positivity is actually far easier than you may think. I don't have numbers to back that up, but it's got to be over 50 percent. This is due in large part due to the fact that for those who don't live in the shadows. Positivity is cool, but if you're in the trenches, hand-to-hand fighting, positivity could mean the difference between life and death. But what is a positive mental attitude (PMA) and how do you get one? Well, I'm glad you asked, a PMA is easy to explain, not as easy to put in action, but well worth the effort. PMA is a philosophy requiring the devotee to have an optimistic outlook, to actively seek the silver lining and consider all of the small joys that surround us daily. But wait, if you act in the next fifteen minutes, I will double the offer, that's right, you will get twice the positivity, twice the joy. Your spouse will start talking to you again, your kids will stop calling you creepy, and your dog will stop biting your crotch. No, it's not that easy; nothing worthwhile really ever is. You have to rewire some technical big word stuff in your brain, which, as any well-educated lab coat wearer would tell you, ain't no picnic on the banks of the Seine during the high season.

Depression sufferers are used to negativity. It feels like home, a horrible home with Velcro toilet paper and basic cable, but home just the same. It is comfortable not because we love it but because it makes sense to us; for some strange reason, it feels real. Since this is the case, it is where we always go back to when we find ourselves on uneven footing or in a complex or confusing situation. The first thing that you must do is believe in your capacity to have a positive thought. You may think I'm being funny—believe me, I'm not funny, at all. The efficacy of PMA is solely reliant on your ability to believe that you, in fact, can say or do something positive in nature. This is important. You have to want to do it. This isn't Viagra that you take, hoping it doesn't last too long, you know, because there's stuff to watch on TV. This is something requiring positive input and action. That, my friends, is how it starts, one positive act performed meaningfully, which then will lead to another, and before you know it, your home just got a little brighter.

The first major hurdle you may find is that when you have the opportunity to be positive, you just don't feel like it, and that quick it's gone like three boxes of Tagalongs she should have hidden better. Instead of feeling worse for missing an opening, try this, smile. There has been a lot of studies done that conclude that smiling, even when you're not happy will improve your mood, and lower your stress and anxiety. This is due to a powerful chemical reaction in your brain that releases tiny molecules called neuropeptides and other neurotransmitters like dopamine and serotonin that have pain relieving and antidepressant qualities. It also raises your midi-chlorian count, possibly giving you the ability to choke people and lift shit with your mind. Remember that the sources for all this information are stored at a place called Google, so call them on the phone with any questions. So the deal is, smile, smile even if you don't want to, smile especially if you don't want to, smile like your trying to sell a crappy camper to an old lady, then when your brain is high on neurotransmitters and shit, smile harder. Never underestimate the power that a simple smile can have or what it can lead to, so after you smile, no matter how hard it is or how fraudulent you may feel in the effort, keep it up and then be open and receptive to what follows. Being a positive influence is as much about the small things is big so say something nice, help someone with their bags, throw a quarter in an expired meter, and just allow humane to become a part of human. Lastly, this is a vital step, so don't skip it, when you've done, said, or thought something positive, make a big deal of it, lift yourself up, go buy an ice cream, and throw some peanut butter and sprinkles on that bitch. Better yet, tell someone, take the win, enjoy it, then build on it.

Work through the feeling of disingenuousness. I know everyone puts an emphasis on genuineness, but most people wouldn't know genuine if it cut off their leg and put it in a wood chipper, so go ahead, fake it until you make it. Chances are, if you're anything like me, you won't know when the faking ends and the making begins, and that is kind of the point. No matter where you are, no matter how dark, how deep down the rabbit hole, just give it a go. Believe me when I say your depression isn't going anywhere, and it just may change your life. Imagine being on a surfboard, enjoying your day, looking cool to nonsurfers with your deep tan and white stuff on your nose, when suddenly a shark eats your fucking arm off! Would you find yourself in a dark place? How would you recover? That very thing happened to Bethany Hamilton, and do you know how she answered those questions? Through the power of positive thinking and force of will, she worked her way back to the surfboard and back to surfing. If I was on a surfboard and a shark took a picture of my arm, I would shit myself, then move to Nebraska, in that order. What it illustrates, however, is the undisputed power of positivity and the unmistakable benefit of positive thoughts and actions, given a chance it can redefine what is possible in your life and the lives of those you touch.

FRIDAY, JULY 3, 2020

This morning Lisa and I decided to go to the gym for an early class, so after getting up, making the bed, taking the "hounds of hell-o" around the block, we head out to get our shirts wet. Before leaving, we got the coffee all ready to go, so Noah's one job when he woke up was to push the go button and that delightful simmering bean water will be awaiting our return like the longing heart of a lovelorn betrothed.

You know by now my goal since my "mental setback," or if you prefer my "falling of the reality wagon," has been to portray a level of transparency in my life. To illuminate the things, I have done and am doing, both positive and negative, with the hopes that it will inspire others who may be struggling to do something, not to do something, or at least begin a mental dialogue about your depression. I've been walking through this less-friendly Tim Burton movie for a long, long time and am still upright and taking solids. I tell you this honestly, I don't think that there is anything you can do for yourself, outside meds and therapy, that is any better for you than exercise. I know, believe me, when someone says exercise, half the people say, "Oh shit, here we go with the lecture," while the other half say, "Yeah, bro, I got this." I'm just going to talk about my experience, and you can take it or leave it, but it's stuff I've got to say.

Of course I first feel compelled and moved by the spirits of litigations past, present, and future to mention first and foremost that I'm not a doctor or a person who knows stuff, so if your highest activity output is getting out of that you shaped indention on the couch, and you know I've been there, first have a medico give you a

78

once-over and clear you for duty. Three, two, one, beep. I used to be a person who would comfort himself with food. On more than one occasion, I have eaten so much, put such a volume of food into my body, that I threw up, which is stupid and super gross because of the sheer volume of all the stuff that comes out. Food is such a psychological fixation in our lives. We remember the times we were hungry. We emotionalize the times food was a part of good memories and bad. Family get-togethers with fun and laughter but also cake and ice cream, picnics with chips, hot dogs, and piecakies, pie stuffed with cake, which has been stuffed with cookies. I grew up in house where it was a requirement to eat more than you needed to, and it was as much social as it was nutritional.

So I would eat, then feel bad because I looked bad, which fed my depression, which was treated by injecting comfort food directly into my mouth, which made me feel worse, which fed my depression, and so it went just an unhappy chubby guy and his bloated depression. The heaviest I officially weighed was three hundred and twenty-four pounds, which was before my last "bender" where I ate everything including *Ficus* leaves and packing peanuts, because I heard peanut. So let's just agree that I was three hundred thirty pounds because it's a nice round number. Let me say this before I go any farther. I in no way want to demonize any body shape or how much anyone weighs. No matter where you are, if you're happy and feel good, then love your life and revel in it. I felt bad about my weakness, about how I looked and how low my self-esteem was, and sure, some of that may have been fueled by the superficial biases of today's mainstream media, but I wasn't where I wanted to be physically, mentally, or emotionally.

Over the years I have started a hundred diets and exercise routines. I did it for my wife or my kids, and each time I would attach just a little more shame and guilt to the burden I carried, which, if life was fair, would have at least a little aerobic value to it. Nothing really stuck until I got to the point where I realized that if I don't do this for myself, I'm not going to do it, so I watched the film on all my previous failures and made a plan. First, I'm not going to start on a fucking Monday. It's so cliché. I'm going to start on Tuesday.

The next thing is that I'm not doing all or nothing anymore, no cold turkeys running around, no going from couch to Olympic marathon podium in a week. This time I'm going to start with small goals over time. I'm going to measure my progress over a year, not a week.

I ate the same food. If I was mashing up Ho-Hos into a dip for my chips, then I continued, making sure, however, to just eat a little less. At the same time, I started walking. My first day I walked a mile. The next day I would eat just a little less and walk just a little more. Each day I laced up I would walk the same route just to the next streetlight before turning around. I have learned that streetlights on the same side of the street are about two hundred and fifty feet apart, and if you increase your distance by this amount each day, it will take around twenty days to add another mile to your daily effort. Each day I did an "eat less, walk more" combo, I did something I had never done before—I took the victory, and I allowed myself to enjoy the win, and positive self-reinforcement felt damn good.

I made quick gains. Soon I had cut my food intake in half and was starting to substitute higher nutritional value items for the processed, homogenized large-breed-dog crap I was eating. At the same time, I had made it to the three-mile mark on my walks, so I began carrying a backpack, empty at first, then each day I would add a small item to it, just a little weight, again over time, adding a little intensity, preparing my joints for what was to come. Time to get preachy. For the love of Tony Little's Gazelle, don't scrimp on shoes. Buy the best shoes you can afford. More-expensive shoes are that way because they are made of better stuff, especially the foam support, which is absolutely something you need, and replace them more frequently than you financially want to. The crap you take from your wallet will be drowned out by the praise your joints sing to your wisdom and leadership.

I progressed steadily over time, going from backpack to jog/walk, to the jog, to the run, to the gym. Over that time, I suffered setbacks in both diet and exercise, which is common to the human condition. I hate to use a social media, pop culture term "trending," because I'm not that hip, but you need to have an understanding that eating a whole cake one day or forsaking the gym for a hammock strung between palm trees is not a problem as long as your week and month is trending in the right direction. Do not put pressure on yourself to be perfect. First, it's impossible. Second, there was only one perfect person ever, and look what happened to him.

Over the past five years of continued improvement, winning, losing, crying, and sweating, I have lost almost one hundred fifty pounds, have cleaned up my diet significantly, and have completely removed the psychological stimulus that I once attached to food. Again, this is not about negating the value of food or to taint the relationship you have with it. It's not about getting likes for the douchebag bathroom selfie *after* picture. My life's journey has been about maximizing what I've been given, about not settling for merely existing, when so much more is possible. I was not comfortable in my own skin, and I wouldn't wish that on anyone.

Exercise has been a vital to the management of my weight, my mental attitude, and closely related, my depression. My overall health and mood have improved, my self-confidence is up, and as far as my depression goes, often the sweatier I get, the cleaner I feel. There is a cautionary tale somewhere hidden between the lines of text about looking good and feeling good. Every good thing can be taken bad levels. Too much masturbation will make you blind. Too little, coincidentally, will make you cross-eyed and angry. Exercise overdone can lead to its own place of dominance over your life, wear your body down to the point of injury, and make you a preworkout-drinking, spandex-wearing, macro-counting nutbag, so do yourself and people who love you a favor, listen to your mind and body and keep it healthy.

Today's daily meditation was utterly custom-tailored for what we just talked about. It was a quick study on the difference between resolutions and intentions. From my comfortable seated position with relaxed posture, hands folded in my lap and intentionally connected breathing, I learned that resolutions are made to deal with what we deem as our negative characteristics, such as being overweight or lacking ambition, and that the solution is based on structured rigid confines. One may tell oneself, "I'm going to go to the gym five days a week," "I'm going to stop eating desert after every meal," or "I'm going to get a job that pays actual money, not crypt-o-moolah." Given the set parameters, at the first failure the whole venture goes out the window. Resolutions put pressure on us to perform to a certain level, a level we obviously will be challenged to meet. Where there is pressure, there is stress, and depression is sure to be lurking nearby.

Intention, on the other hand, is far kinder and has inherent flexibility allowing for the reality that is human nature. "I intent to live a healthier, more active life" allows you to work through the improvement process without the pressure of perfection hanging over your head like a constipated pigeon. So this New Year, when someone asks what you resolution is, tell them "to make a sombrero out of actual human skin and tissue," then give them a creepy smile and ask them what kind of lotion they use. Therefore, be compassionate to yourself, set an intention not a resolution, and remember, small changes over time make a big difference. If you sail out of New York on a course heading of ninety degrees, eventually you will hit Portugal. By adjusting your course less than 1 percent, or five degrees, it will put you off the coast of Western Sahara, Africa, over twelve hundred miles away from Portugal, which would lead to questions about you seafaring skills if indeed you were trying to reach Portugal. This is, of course, a double-edged sword as small negative changes over time can have opposite effects and lead to a very unhappy you.

It's all about you. I know we train ourselves to put others first. We are taught from an early age to not be selfish, and this works against us in so many ways as we move through life. We need to understand that by taking on the responsibility of putting our interests in the spotlight, then we are taking care of our families and those around us by proxy. I know, people everywhere cite the preflight safety briefing about putting your mask on before assisting others, and also don't smoke in the lavatory. While I get that, I don't see it that way. In an emergency, survival takes priority and precedence. For me, it's wearing a life jacket on a fishing trip. When you take control of your own safety and well-being, not only are your actions teaching self-importance and respect, but should an emergency arise, you are prepared and ready. Let that sink in for a moment. By making you stronger physically and mentally, you are taking care of the things that are important in your life. Now let this slap you across the face. What does it mean if you are not taking care of yourself?

I honestly believe in my heart that if I can do something, then a discarded breath mint can do it as well. Despite what my mother always told me, there is nothing special about me that would allow me to do anything that couldn't be replicated given time and effort. You want to climb a mountain, dive with sharks, make love on an active erupting volcano just for the double entendre? You do not have to allow anything in your life to hold you back from being the best version of yourself, and that includes you, my friend.

Saturday, July 4, 2020

When you get up in the middle of the night, do you check to see what time it is? Follow up question, do you still own an alarm clock? I haven't owned an alarm clock in what feels like decades, but in reality, it's probably been seven or eight years. I never really trusted it either. Some nights I would stare at the red digital numbers, just knowing it was waiting for the most important meeting of my financial year to secure its revenge for my years of hard pushing its tiny sensitive plastic buttons. "Revenge is a dish best served late, bitch." I don't want to know what time it is when I pinball my way back down the hall, eyes barely open to prevent synapses from firing, doing everything possible to tell my brain it's still asleep. "It's only midnight, still much sleepy, sleepy time." The deal is, it may be around midnight, or it may be around four in the morning, which would break my heart and leave me lying there thinking about how I would get Lisa to salute the idea of a bedroom urinal that I hoisted up the flagpole.

On most days, I'm up and going a minimum of three hours before necessity would merit. Nonetheless, my actions are built about depression management, and by getting up as I do, my depression doesn't have a say in the decision. Like I mentioned earlier, I see my depression as not a part of me but not as another person either. This is often the part of the story where people's eyes squint a little and their heads tilt slightly as if they were dogs and you said "treat." My depression is a stand-alone ghoulish, dark being that is never far away and is always scheming and plotting. It's like the movie "the Grudge" but real, and not Japanese, not that there's any wrong with Japan; I'm sure their depression is fine. The advantage of knowing my depression the way that I do is that I can predict and counter areas where attacks may be imminent. Mornings can be an issue, so I remove the opportunity by just getting up and getting moving.

Speaking of moving, this morning is another early workout class we scheduled earlier in the week when it sounded like a way better idea than it does at the moment. What I really want to do right now is sit down with my dark, rich, hot cup and enjoy the summer sunrise, but discipline builds character, or some shit like that, so I put my gym clothes on and head down the hall to get the coffee ready for later.

The temporary regret I felt earlier for scheduling an early morning sweat sesh is replaced by a feeling of achievement and relief as we head home to plan the day and have a cup of amazingness, and yes, I have it under control, I could quit any time, and I just choose not to, ever. As with most Saturdays, Noah and I will head to the grocery store before hungry hordes follow, allowing us the freedom to shop the aisles in any fucking direction we so choose. Take that, the man. Around our house, we like to pitch in and do chores as a team, and every team has a superstar. Lisa is our Michael Jordan. She, honestly, does the most and runs the show. We're just here because they had extra uniforms and because, every once in a while, even Michael, I mean Lisa, has got to pass the ball. We follow her lead and support her the best we can, by putting away laundered and folded clothes, taking out garbage and recycling, peeling her off the rogue blackberry bushes that are taking over our backyard like a thorny green land kraken.

Josh is coming for a visit per usual, so later I will be staring down the barrel of my PTSD once again, and while the bathroom plumbing repair is holding, I've noticed more and more being put down the garbage disposal in the kitchen, which doesn't bode well. That being said, I feel much more at ease today than I did one week ago, and I attribute this to my daily practice of meditation and contemplation. It would seem that even my most novice of attempts are making a very real difference, and when something that was "mystic" in my mind works as advertised, I get all tingly in my nethers.

For the first time in, I don't know five or six months I'm not experiencing anxiety about Josh coming over. This is such a huge difference from even last week, where stress was present but not over-powering. I am even breaking one of my rules, even though it was a temporary rule written with crayon on a Post-it note and stuck to my frontal lobe. I am thinking about J Man's outing at our house, where before it was a no-no because even thinking about it got the blood pressure up a bit. I am doing something right, and it has imbued me with hope that a degree of control over my PTSD, and overall angst is ultimately possible. Another novel sensation that I am experienc-ing is a pleasant anticipation of my upcoming therapy session with Dr. K on the ninth. So many dreaded sessions where I couldn't wait for the beep of timer that signaled my torture was over for the day and someone else's would soon start. Now I'm a little boy excited to take his fluffy puppy to show and tell.

There is so much more for me to learn about this meditation thing, and I've just begun to walk down this path. I know that taking advice from me in this arena is like learning the art of vegan cooking from Hannibal Lecter, but I can go over my experience, and you can take it with a grain of salt, and maybe a nice Chianti. Keeping in mind that I have no training whatsoever and receive my input from my phone/alarm clock, I find it even more fascinating that it works so well for me. I see meditation and contemplation are separate but closely related, like when that lovable redneck introduces you to his sister-fiancée.

I have found that for me, I get more "om" for the buck when I meditate then contemplate. I use the meditation as a mental warm-up, a cerebral stretch and limbering session, getting ready for the contemplation that will follow. Something you probably don't know about me is that I hate prepping for almost anything. I don't like stretching more than twelve seconds before working out, food prep is limited to making the food directly before I eat it, and if you want something painted and it requires masking, your better be a Pollack fan, 'cause shits fix'n to get all splatty up in here. I mention this for no other reason than to pat myself on the back and tell you that you're never too old to get better.

John Wayne once said in a movie that "a man's got to know his limitations," and I believe everything he ever said like "slap some bacon on a biscuit, and let's go!" That being the case, I cannot yet do meditation on my own. It's still difficult for me to center and focus my mind and control my breathing without cues or instructions. My mind still wants to chase squirrels and hump legs, but my leash is now much shorter, making bringing myself back to focus much faster and easier. Using the "daily calm" app on my phone really enables my freshness to this discipline by leading me through daily short get-togethers that encompass focus, breathing, and a topic of meditation that lead me into contemplation. That's a great endorsement. Someone should be paying me to say shit like that, at least a gift basket with assorted crackers and jams from around the world.

The other day the "calm" topic was marshmallows and revolved around a study of four-year-olds at Stanford University. The kids were offered a delicious marshmallow that they could eat immediately, or if they agreed to wait fifteen minutes, they could have two. Seventy percent of the children chose the instant gratification over waiting. Even more interesting I found is that they revisited the children fifteen years after the experiment concluded to study if any difference between the two groups could be ascertained. What was found was that the group that chose to wait were healthier, happier, and more successful on average than the group choosing to partake immediately, which led to the takeaway of taking time to think on a decision reduces urges that could be detrimental to a person's health and financial well-being. I would have put that white fluffy son of a bitch in my mouth so fast I would have been tasting researcher fingers. I always ask the question "How would this relate to my depression or my life?" With this topic, I feel that it's just a reaffirmation to not act on impulse, to take a mindful approach to decision-making and explore all known options and ramifications, and marshmallows are best consumed almost on fire with chocolate and graham crackers.

Deep breath, back to center, good. I know you have a question about breathing, and I'm with you. I thought it was automatic too, just set it and forget it, but there is so much more to breathing than sucking and blowing. I know that sounds dirty, but I'm going to let it stand. Focused breathing techniques are way more about the mind than the breath. It's about leaving the hustle and bustle of your life, the constant tug-of-war with your attention, where breath slows you down and pays your toll to cross the border into a state of mindfulness. If you're looking for a ten-thousand-foot view of what mindfulness is, seek it elsewhere. I'm on the runway flapping cardboard wings, but I'll tell you what I think mindfulness is. Mindfulness is simply bringing special awareness to the things all around us that we experience each day, but we are too busy to notice or simply take them for granted. Breathing affects so much in our lives and bodies, has more elements than you would ever know, by bringing a hyperawareness and understanding to the breathing, and allows you mind to see and experience the whole world differently. Details become clearer, and we gain understanding of issues where once clarity eluded us. This is why I use breathing and meditation to lead me into contemplation.

While still focused on intentional breathing and with a present but subdued mind, I begin to contemplate and open the mental file drawer labeled "depression shit" and see what emerges. I find it utterly fascinating what issues arise during this phase of my process, but stuff from decades ago comes to my mind but with a clarity that I never experienced before. I have put more unresolved issues to their final rest over the past week than in the entirety of my overall existence. When I was in the Air Force, I had a dear friend that I thought the world of. When we were off duty, our families would spend some evenings and weekends together, mostly doing stuff that didn't cost a lot of money since we were all poor. He was married to a wonderful lady, and together they had a beautiful baby daughter. Lisa had Mack, I don't know, a year or so before, so we made the perfect group. That all changed one day when he went on a temporary duty assignment, three weeks overseas, no big deal, unless you start up a relationship with a human enjoyment service provider and take and bring home photographic evidence of said liaison, as a souvenir? Once the truth came out, we did the best we could to support each of them, but the die had been cast, they separated, and he took the first overseas gig he could get. I bring this up for the reason that this incident happened over two decades ago, but it really bothered me, and

I had not processed it, just pushed it down to move forward. Don't make it weird, but when he cheated on his wife, I felt like he cheated on all of us, and I was hurt. I realize that now, I was able to achieve a level of understanding and acceptance, and it was like a case closed.

Keeping in mind that I'm still an infant blowing baby powder farts when it comes to this, but I am seeing and more importantly feeling results. I feel overall more centered during the day and haven't experienced any PTSD issues so far, and Josh has been here for a few hours now. He has been very industrious today, shredding various random things like books and punching bag gloves, which sucks because I use them, especially when I punch a bag. I don't know if I've ever talked about his shredding, but it's something he enjoys, and it's just like it sounds. He takes stuff and with his fingers and teeth makes it into much smaller stuff. He then throws it out of his bathroom window, through the screen that he ripped a hole in for that solitary purpose. He used to want to throw it over the fence into the neighbor's yard, which is great because giving people junk is an amazing way to foster goodwill; we were able to break him of that habit by planting some tall shrubs that block him from getting close enough. We keep a variety of items in his room, ranging from cardboard to foam, books, and VHS tapes, just in case the mood arises, just another piece to the "this is why we can't have nice stuff" puzzle.

As it is my fashion, I have spoken far too soon. When Lisa was getting Josh ready to go home, she was trying to clip his fingernails, and he got upset. He let out this guttural irritated grunt that I have heard a thousand times, but it set me off like a donkey kick to the dick, a dick kick. My stomach turned, and I became flushed and sweaty. The room seemed to move independent of my body as I felt my heart race well past the aerobic zone. I was in full on PTSD mode, and making it to the living room chair was a challenge. I sat there for what seemed like an hour. Lisa the all-knowing, understanding what was going on, tried to comfort me by getting Joshua ready to transition from our house back to his own, removing the J variable from the equation. By the time he was ready, I was able to walk him out and get him buckled in. I know he sensed my emotional distress as I kissed his forehead. He looked at me, a rare occurrence, and I told him I love him and am proud of him, then made my way back to my seat. I tried to center myself but was unable, still too fresh, couldn't rein in my mind.

I just sat taking purposeful breaths, breathing in and breathing out for what seemed like a long time. Lisa hadn't returned, so it couldn't have been more than fifteen twenty minutes, but over that time, life had slowly returned to normal. I got up and busied myself with straightening the big man's room for his return the following week. The anxiety was gone by the time Lisa pulled in the driveway. She sat a moment in her car, pondering I guess whether she wanted to come in and what state she would find me in. Her brow relaxed a bit when she realized that I hadn't gone catatonic and that I had worked through the situation to a functional degree. We talked about it, not to great depth, neither of us wanting to cross any unseen trip-wires that might cause relapse.

It is clear to me that I had become overconfident. I had experienced a degree of success, and I allowed it to create a sense of security that had not been earned through time and effort. I had manufactured my own Maginot line, fabricated it with naivety and optimism, much like the one in France, and had seen it ravaged in moments, again, historically accurate. Today a valuable lesson was learned, one that I fear I have learned before about overconfidence and underestimation, revisited in different stages of my life around different circumstances, but of value nonetheless. My excitement about my upcoming session with Dr. K has been tarnished by this recent bout of PTSD. I wanted to be the monkey with a new trick, but maybe this little setback was exactly what I needed to keep me focused on improving.

It's ironic, I think, that I'm dealing with PTSD on a day when so many others will experience it in varying degrees as the sun heads west and darkness takes hold. This year, given the 'Rona and event restrictions in place, all big fireworks displays had been canceled, meaning that citizens were left to their own devices when it came to blowing shit up to celebrate the birthday of America, which is never ideal. News reports detailed record sales in consumer fireworks from the hastily built county-fair-esque stands that pop up on roadsides, and given that our state forbids fireworks that fly, all we got is loud and high-pitched obnoxious whistley fountains going off in salvos far past bedtime. I have new found respect for anyone having to deal with PTSD and understanding why it can be such a big deal. I've had it for only a short time and would rather skydive naked into a burning thumbtack factory than go through that again.

My recovering mind shifts gears to when I was a kid, I almost set a neighbor's house on fire by creating my own firework made from sparklers and duct tape. So not to find myself on a list at some government agency, I won't go into detail, but when lit, these improvised firework devices would either explode dramatically or take off dramatically. Of course, safety is on the list, so I always had a bucket of water somewhere in my vicinity just in case, but again, I felt confident in my pyrotechnic ability having never really burnt anyone to death, so I kept building bigger and boomier. I lit this particularly large model I called ominously the enchanted death blossom and stood back to be entertained. The thrill I felt as the blossom took flight was quickly replaced with dread as I watched it streak toward the neighbor's house like a laser-guided scud missile. Thoughts of smoking cigs on the yard at juvie, trying to not get shivved, crossed my mind as I was sure it was going to crash through a window and explode into flames, killing the poor family who resided within its walls. At the last moment, call it fate, or God, or just a sudden gust of wind, but the flying flaming death hit the eaves and thudded to the ground, catching on fire. I hurdled the fence like I was running that one hurdle race and quickly doused it, rendering it harmless, and giving me my freedom back, on Independence Day.

If this was any other year, we would have been at the ballpark, watching minor league baseball followed by a big firework display that I would leave early from, you know, to beat all of the other suckers home. I would have eaten a hot dog and maybe an ice cream sundae out of a small baseball helmet. After all, it is America's birthday. As it turns out, we'll probably start yawning as the sun goes down and end up in bed early, comforting three shivering dogs from the "purge" happening just outside our walls.

God, I hate assholes. I get staying up late and setting off fireworks that sparkle and make loud noises and that it only really gets good after your seventh cheap beer when you start lighting fireworks with other lit fireworks because you can no longer hold the match steady. There is, however, no call whatsoever for setting off an atomic comet super fountain at three o'clock in the ante meridiem. After literally smelling the napalm in the morning, I lay there thinking of my episode yesterday, feeling still overall positive about the direction I'm heading and the progress I've made. I tell myself "PTSD is thoughts and thoughts can be controlled." Just keep working. Don't give up. I haven't yet. I get up and get the coffee going.

This morning we are making the two-and-a-half-hour drive south down the interstate to visit with Bill and Nancy. Bill's condition has steadily declined, and we want to visit and help Nancy where and how we can. It's been a little while since seeing him, and I feel a sense of unease about the trip that I just can't seem to put my finger on, but my coffee comforts me like a helicopter mom on a rough day, so I keep sipping. I will probably drink too much today.

I know what you're thinking and your right, to a degree. Addiction is a study in fine lines until it isn't. I don't know what scientific percentage of correlation between depression and addiction is, but I know that there has been a lot of studies done, and I would assume that the number is high. I would look it up, but then my computer thinks that I have a problem and will forever show me counseling advertisements. When someone is both addicted and depressed the treatment for each is exponentially complicated. It's like having to drive across Los Angeles at rush hour but first drinking a gallon of colonoscopy prep.

While I am not prone to addiction (caffeine notwithstanding), I am addiction adjacent. I've never taken drugs, and by drugs I mean if you can't buy it with a debit card in front of your mother talking to a priest, then it's a drug. I believe that I have always understood their capacity to destroy all they touch, having known personal examples of this in my life. If I'm being honest, and I like to think I am usually over 50 percent. I have never ever had a person offer me drugs or a circumstance where I had to say no. I think my strict policy of not knowing any drug dealers, pushers, or mules have really paid dividends.

Alcohol, however, is another matter entirely. In the not too distant past I drank, and I'm not just talking about "Hey, let's grab a beer." I'm talking about all-out, no-holds-barred, unadulterated shit-facedness. I drank socially, then to have fun, then for the demons, then to dull the pain and anguish of living with demons, then to get so drunk I would engage in activities that would facilitate my demise. I have a friend who lives in a neighborhood on a steep winding hill. I once got drunk and rode my bike home, barreling down the serpentine lane, traveling forty-five miles an hour, tears from the wind racing across my cheeks. I deftly maneuvered around obstacles, weaving through traffic, making my way across town just like Kevin Bacon in that bike movie, but drunk off my ass. I was the greatest, nondoping cyclist alive until about a half mile from home around a gentle curve on the bike path, I unexpectedly left the path and hit a maple tree.

I would drink a little at home from time to time, but as I understand the rules, if you drink alone at home, you're an alcoholic, whereas if you get self-embalmed at a social gathering, you're just "fun." So I would look for events or create ones with the sole purpose of generating an opportunity or reason to celebrate some random thing, and then I would do my thing, and by my thing I mean I would "pre-funk" drinking several beverages before the event for marination, then drink hard and fast until I reached that glorious level of "Did I piss my pants, or am I currently pissing my pants?" I would do this as often as I could get away with it. Again, the rules are clear. If you get drunk every week, alcoholic.

Clearly I was indulging in extreme behavior, and with extreme behavior comes consequences, repercussions, and sometimes a free portrait session from the local jail, which luckily I've avoided because of my desire to one day be pope because of the hat. I began to see a change in my overall demeanor, and my behavior became more and more erratic. I began to feel a compulsion, a tug toward the bottle that would start midweek and increase as the weekend neared. I began to find some of the weight that I worked diligently to lose, of course from the alcohol, but also from the inebriation induced inhibitions that made everything seem more delicious. "Do you know what would be great on nachos? Pie!" If you're wondering where Lisa was during this whole unfurling of Rodger period, she stood right behind me, with her foot as far up my ass if she could cram it. I was a constant irritation, and she used all tools at her disposal—understanding, guilt, disappointment, and anger, hoping to adjust my decision-making paradigms. If there was a Norwegian committee that met annually and awarded a prize to the person who has lived with a difficult spouse while displaying grace, courage, and leadership, Lisa would make it to the podium, bronze for sure.

There is a time when an issue achieves critical mass, when a decision must be made that will address the issue or allow it unhindered to develop into a problem. I passed that time, but then I went back and acted like I hadn't. I knew that I, once again, had to make a change in my life and, of course, if you can't make a change to your behavior when you know you have to, you're an alcoholic. Change is hard, I'm not going to lie, especially when you tie some good times with friends and events and experiences you've loved. It's even harder with alcohol, because it's harder to ween yourself off, especially at first. You just can't say, "I'm only going to have eight beers instead of ten" because honestly after five you start to think that banana is a number. The first couple of weeks were the hardest. I didn't have withdrawals or get the shakes, but there was definitely a tug, a yearning that had to quelled. I picked the right time on my calendar given I didn't have any social engagements planned, which gave me the opening to go without, while not feeling deprived of social engagement or just plain fun. My depression flared as I stepped away from something I believed was important to my treatment. I know now that the depression wanted the addiction. It fed it and nurtured it by feigning defeat while I was under the influence, making me feel that what I was doing was in some weird way beneficial, which is diabolical if you think about it.

I didn't do anything to "kick" alcohol but suffer and work, putting time between me and the bottle, the more time, the less I wanted it in my life. I do, to this day, miss some of the elements of those days, that point when all is seems right with a world on fire, when even stupid stuff like riding your bike into a dumpster would make you laugh, but I think what I miss most is the drunk plans I would make with drunk friends. I planned trips around the world to see some of the Google screensavers, I've started a Fortune 500 company that created dissolvable underwear, and I've solved half of the world's problems using a watermelon-throwing trebuchet. I've also lost a connection with some people who I thought were friends that just wanted drunk company, and that always hurts, but it always happens.

I haven't had a drink in five months at this point, and while I'm confident that I could without it leading to another, I found that I seem to have lost the taste for it. I no longer crave a beer on a hot day. The thought of a glass of wine makes me long for the day of sucking soap because I said "poontang" around my mom, whatever that meant, and even the thought of my favorite, gin and tonic, creates no excitement.

Now I know that addiction goes beyond altering substances. Practically everything can be taken to the extreme; food, shopping, tattoos and piercings, German fetish porn, and even religion can be taken to that elevated place in our lives. If something makes you feel good and takes away your focus from pain and suffering, it has the capacity for addiction. Even healthy things like exercising, drinking water, and oral coffee enemas can lead to fixations and dysmorphia, which render them useless and unhealthy. If you are a depression sufferer, there is an even greater risk than just becoming an addict.

Understanding that your depression will entangle itself within the emotional strata of your dependence, building control as you lose it. I'm sure that you've heard the story of the two wolves that live within you where one is positive and the other negative, or one is good and one is bad, or one parallel parks nose first and the other leads with its ass. Either way, the answer to question of which one is stronger is always answered the same way—it's the one you feed. In my version, there's just you and the wolf, and if you're getting weaker, who's getting stronger? It was a rhetorical question; it's the wolf. So always be aware of and honest about who's getting dinner based on your thoughts, feelings, and actions.

Now that I've given my lecture and feel pretty good about myself, it's time to fill up my travel mug with something hot and creamy and get buckled up for our trip down the freeway. I make it the better part of twenty minutes before my right ass cheek needs a good kneading from someone with significant grip strength. An hour later, I've fully reverted to my twelve-year-old self wondering "When the poontang are we going to be there?" This is absolutely why I don't do road trips anymore. If I have to sit, I would rather sit faster, like at five hundred miles per hour. Traffic is light, and despite my posterior discomfort, we make good time.

In the lulls of conversation, my mind would constantly land on what we were heading toward. I have been around people fighting for their very lives, and I have been there when they lost that fight. It always takes a toll on everyone involved, the living and the dying. Our mission is to lift Bill and Nancy's spirits as much as we can, help where it's needed, and just share some time together. When someone passes, it's the little things that are most missed, like sitting around a table and talking about nothing and everything or strolling together along a path after a spring rain shower.

We pulled in almost to the minute when we told them to expect us, which always brings a brief moment of satisfaction. Nancy noticed our arrival and met us outside on the front porch, where we exchanged hugs and headed into the house. We had all donned masks prior to getting out of the car, which has become a ritual that I still can't quite get accustomed to, always feeling more felonious than hospitable, like we're here to visit, but also to steal any pastries you may have. We entered and greeted Bill, obeying whatever protocol we believed governed situations such as these, and kept our distance and masks until Bill gave the cue that it was acceptable to remove them. He looked good and had shaved the mustache that had resided on his upper lip since I had known him. Bill sat uneasy in his easy chair as if he was contemplating something or trying to find the words that would properly explain what he was experiencing.

Noticing the struggle, we talked about the weather, then fireworks, then the not-so-temporary insanity that the world has been experiencing as of late. Soon his easy smile had found its way back to his face, and it was just like old times, human beings being human, laughing, remembering, every moment bittersweet. Death has always interested me, not in a morbid vampirism fixation but in the sway it holds over the living. The fear and realization of loss has such raw power to control our lives. It motivates like nothing else and produces unmatched joy or profound heartbreak. So many times I longed for the restful embrace that death offered that I saw a person's passing as a blessing, an end to their earthly pain and suffering. I know that not all deaths are equal, just as not all lives are equal. Some deaths seem to be rewards for living good lives and fighting hard until the end, while others feel much more tragic, men, women, boys, and girls passing suddenly, far before their time, and far beyond our understanding, leaving voids in the lives of all they touched.

It is no wonder that death is the dominion of depression. It revels in bereavement, rejoices in the torment that it produces. It is the darkest vulture that feeds on the living. For many, their first experience with depression will be a result of a loved ones passing to the other side. For most it will pass; the darkness will not take hold and linger after the mourning and closure is achieved. For others the seed will find fertile soil and it will grow, becoming part of that person's existence following its prime directive—kill the host and perpetuate itself in others. If you are grieving, I am sorry for your loss and pain. I hope that you will hold your cherished memories close to your heart remembering the good times and laughter. Do not despair, avoid anger and hatred, strive to find a degree of acceptance, and be on vigilant guard with the understanding that your loved one would not want their passing to lead to yours.

As our visit continued, Bill's eyelids started to lose their battle with gravity, so we took that as a cue to take our leave. We gave long hugs and smiles, hoping that our eyes would say all the important things we thought better of saying out loud, hoping Bill and Nancy understood that sometimes words are the poorest representation of how we really feel. We drive away, hoping that there will be more time and that we can do this again soon. My heart feels heavy in my chest, my mind rewinding and replaying the last time I saw my mom. I sighed. "Jesus, I need a coffee!"

This morning hit me like naked blackberry harvesting, unpleasant on so many levels. For the first time in a while I really wanted to say, "Fuck the fray, I'm staying in bed!" Stupid fucking wolf subcontext sprinkled throughout my life. My mind told me, "We are the sum of what we create." I don't know what the hell that means, but it sounds important, so I got my ass up and make the bed taking special care to ensure that it's perfect, that the corners are equal and symmetrical, that there are no visible wrinkles, and that the pillows are properly fluffed with smoothly flattened pillowcases. Short of stroking out, there is no way I'm getting back into this bed until the sun goes down. No retreat today.

The three jumping hairy chalupas were raring to go, behaving like they just downloaded nose upgrades, and it opened up a whole new world of smells that had to be smelled, by smelling everything. We rounded the corner for home and I was ready to be done, the stress of wrangling these air-lickers canceling out the so-called health benefits of spending quality time with your loving pets. This morning will be filled with busy work, a lot of boxes just waiting for a check mark. Lisa and I were going to get our shirts wet, then drop my old battle wagon off for some oily and filtery love, drop off some flyers I created for a socially distancing event, then to the office for emails, faxes, and forms before heading back home.

I am a person of momentum, preferring to move in a direction toward a purpose. Sudden changes or backtracking cuts against my grain something fierce, so when I have places to go or territory to cover, I create a plan that allows me to move as efficiently as possible without going backward. If I forget something along the way, unless it's breathing air or Lisa, I will leave it behind. Sometimes there are casualties. You have to let them go. When I was young, I loved the video game Paper Boy, where you ride your bike down a neighborhood, tossing papers onto the porches of houses, while dodging cars, people, and dogs. You could never go back, so if you missed a house, oh well, if you missed too many houses, you were fired, until the next quarter. I loved this game. Do your job well, get paid, go forward, no going back, ever. In case you were wondering, no, you wouldn't have wanted me delivering your paper. Back in the day, even when we played video games, we were working. Today it's all about exploding heads. Some days I long to go back to when I was twelve, and the world was still filled with wonder and hope.

I remember the day clearly, as if it were last week. It was either the seventh or eighth of July. Actual dates didn't have profound significance to a thirteen-year-old, so if pressed in a court of law, it might have also been the ninth of July 1981. I am, however, not fuzzy one iota about the details that occurred and would confidently raise my hand, put the other on a stack of religious texts that somehow, through magic, compel the truth, and recount the harrowing tale of how I lost my innocence and any hope of a "normal" life.

It was a mild summer day that found me lying on the lush green grass that grew in between the two large apple trees that resided directly behind the garden plot in our backyard. It was the softest, greenest grass on the property, the kind that makes you want to kick off your shoes and let the soft blades tickle the skin in between your toes. I believe that this was the lush, relaxing "garden spot" of the yard because, while my mom ensured that every inch of vegetation received ample watering, this spot, because of the dense foliage of the apple trees, provided relief from the midday sun. I was outside because one of the commandments of my youth was that kids should only be indoors if shelter is required, and since at this moment in time the only form of electric entertainment was three television channels playing soap operas, outside felt like the place to be.

I remember lying on my back, staring up at the blue sky through the mottled latticework of branches, watching the wispy clouds change shapes as they raced from view. It was the kind of day that you wish you could cram into a mason jar, seal up tight with a note to not open until February, and put it in the pantry next to the family-size ketchup and pickled pears that nobody will ever eat unless it's a choice between that and human flesh. I was contented before I knew what it meant or could appreciate it, and it would be the last time I would feel that for the rest of my life. No, that's too dramatic. Let's just say for a long, long time, because what would happen next would change my life forever.

Suddenly, my bright sunny day had darkened as if someone had placed a pumpkin on my head with pantyhose-covered eye holes. I could see. The world just seemed dark and out of focus. I remember feeling lightheaded as my heart tried to beat its way out of my chest. Suddenly I had the feeling that I wasn't alone. I scanned the horizon, squinting then opening my eyes wide, trying to find a clear image of what was before me. I saw the tall friendly cedar trees that lined the property on the east border, then the backside of the house, the picture window that would soon be removed so my dad could build an addition with a leaky roof. The attached carport was empty and devoid of purpose. And lastly, the trellised wine grapes on the western property line held no clues, especially to their purpose since we never consumed them as wine, or grapes for that matter.

I found myself now standing, frozen, wanting to run but not able send the command to my limbs, knowing something was terribly wrong, like when you're in a public bathroom stall and a stranger sits down in the next one over and wants to start up a conversation. Then, suddenly, I caught movement in the covered walkway separating the house proper and carport. Again, my eyes were squinting hard as if the pressure will make them telescope out like in the cartoons and allow me to make out shape and form. I see nothing human, or recognizable, what is before me seems to be a black floating void, about the size of a small child or a large wombat. It hovered motionless about a foot off the ground. My unblinking eyes locked on as my brain struggled to comprehend what was before me. It began to move, slowly, ominously toward me. My skeleton wanted to run, screaming, but my skin and muscle tissue wouldn't allow it, and still it moved closer. It was like a rerun of that *Star Trek* episode with the floating death bot Nomad, where it wanted to kill everyone until Spock mind-melded it to death, but Spock wasn't here, and this thing didn't have a head that I could tell.

I was absolutely terrified. My whole being seemed under control of this malevolent being. I couldn't even piss myself for defensive purposes. Soon it was directly in front of me. I wasn't looking directly at it as much as into it. For lack of better understanding, this was a black hole, an emptiness that seemed to feed off energy all around it. The outer edges of this hovering specter seemed distorted, like it was drawing in the environment around it. I believed that I was next, that I would soon lift off the ground and be sucked into the abyss and out of existence, leaving nothing behind but mystery and my family's sadness. Then something changed, not with the entity, but within me. I felt a sorrow and darkness take a hold of me like I've never experienced before. Hopelessness became a word in my vocabulary, as did despair. Although I was never touched physically by this shadowy wraith, it somehow infected me, poisoned my mind in a profound and mystifying way.

Then, as if accomplishing its mission of evil, it vanished leaving no trace behind. It felt as if I had been under this thing's spell for a long time, fifteen minutes certainly at the least, but time had far less meaning in those days. The sun's brilliance returned, overhead birds chirped and did bird things, the wispy clouds still chased each other across the sapphire sky, and the blades of soft grass still tickled my toes when urged by the cool breeze. It was as if nothing had happened, but I knew deep inside that everything had changed, like I'd seen something that couldn't be unseen, like seeing your mother naked the first time. I found myself able to move but unwilling, preferring to stand there in a state of gobsmackedness, processing information as fast as my tiny little brain could process. I desperately wanted to run to the back door, fling it open, and tell my poor mother everything that just happened, but what had just happened? If a condor swooped down and regurgitated an angry naked leprechaun who promptly took a rainbow-colored dump on your foot before saying

"It's magically delicious," then disappearing, how would you explain that?

When I did move, I didn't run, didn't scream, just walked into the house, passed wordlessly by my busy mom, and headed up the narrow stairway to my stuffy room where I lay on my bed, experiencing my first bout of depression, suffering in silence. That day I claimed a headache as an excuse for my obvious demeanor change and worked through it as best I could, no one the wiser that I had been violated and that the trajectory of my life had been fundamentally altered. I didn't know about depression, or what the word even meant at the time. Back in the day, to learn something about anything we had to go to a library and look stuff up via a card catalog, and everything smelt like soup and grandma's closet. I pieced together my early working knowledge of depression from family stories and experiences with my uncle Jack, but my early days were truly the incompetent leading, well, me. I did know one thing, I was well on my way to becoming Jack. I knew there was something wrong with me, but I was dead set on forcing that wrong onto my parents, so I chose to go it alone, much like Snake Plissken in *Escape from New York*, which is loosely based on my formative years.

That was thirty-nine years ago today, or maybe tomorrow, or day after tomorrow at absolute latest. It is our "lace" anniversary, which is kind of creepy because all I picture is mourning veils around a flower adorned coffin, which is unsettling as fuck. Next year will be our ruby anniversary, and since the ruby was once considered the gem of Ares, god of war, for its red color signifying blood, vengeance, and death, I find it unsettling-er as fuck. No matter, I will mark this occasion and all to come the same way. I will live and strive to be the best, happiest version of myself that is available. I will endeavor to be a centered, positive influence in those around me, and I will never, ever give up. So enjoy our day depression, there will be many more, and oh, I got you this: there's nothing there I'm just holding up my middle finger. I hope you like it.

Tuesday, July 7, 2020

Good morning, how'd you sleep last night? I got some strong, restful hours last night and woke feeling rested, which makes such a difference in the daily headspace beautification process. Lisa rarely goes with me on the morning jaunt around the alps with the miniature nonhelpful St. Bernards, she's usually out running, biking, or climbing Mt. F-ing Everest. When she does join our round the block adventure, the dogs totally lose their shit, each showing off as if trying out for the lead role in *Dogs: The Less Finicky Musical*. If Lisa ever wonders why she doesn't join us more often, that question firmly resides in the "answered" category as we untangle their leads and enter the house.

I really want to talk about the cup of coffee I had in the moments after, but I'm beginning to think that you're quietly judging me. I will say this, that the plantation-grown darkly roasted South American bean is some of the best coffee on earth. Oh, I'm aware that some people might say Kona, or regional Africa, and while I agree they are a full-flavored bean, they are forever being "blended" with inferior beans, which lessens the overall experience and is a real shame. I'll have you know that research has been done on the effects of caffeine and depression, and a positive correlation has been found between coffee intake and overall mood and outlook. The studies found that the effect is greater, or more beneficial, on habitual users, compared with nonconsumers. What this means is that because I'm habitual, my mood is more likely to be brightened by partaking in a hot cup of coffee than some random weirdo who doesn't think coffee as an imperative to life. Oh, still looking for a source? It's far too late in the game to try and add legit-ness by adding credible sources, so I would again tell you to simply call Google.

Today is much like yesterday, a mishmash of errands and service work, a day full of unchecked boxes. First order of business—get the workout done and in the books. From there I need to be dropped off to pick up my truck that had a sleepover with its friends at the garage. I drive a 2007 Nissan Titan pickup that, like its owner, has seen better days physically. It's got dents and scrapes, the seats are decomposing, and if you roll the windows down, you may not get them back up, but it runs good and gets from A to B, and I would park that donkey in a minefield next to a shopping cart emporium, where you need shopping carts to buy shopping carts.

Younger me wouldn't want to be caught in an old beat-up truck. He would have driven it sure, since it was all he could afford, but he wouldn't like it. You see, younger me was a dickhead and cared about image, and nothing showed success like big, shiny, and beyond your means. It didn't help that I'm in a business where the perceived value of what you have to offer is often based on the car you drive, the brand of watch you wear, the insignia embroidered on your shirt, and that your hair has product in it. If depression has done anything beneficial for me, it has been in showing me how stupid superficiality is and how it's not worth ten minutes of darkness, let alone the weeks and months I endured trying to protect my "image."

One thing that you have to know about putting significant emphasis on your image is that it's like a coin. On one side, let's call it heads, is you with your perfectly coifed hair and full Windsor knot imported silk tie. On the other are your insecurities created by tenuous nature of holding the image in place. The bigger the image, the more energy is required to hold it steady. The greater the chance it will crash down around you, the more intense the insecurity. There is nothing that entices depression like insecurity. It's like blood in the water on shark week or chili cheese nachos after a bong session. Depression amplifies insecurity, makes you question your abilities, and makes you doubt your worth, which makes your image even more important. Do you see the vile, vicious nature of this fucking thing? Do you wonder how people find themselves staring down barrels or climbing over bridge railings?

Image is not the sole domain of insecurities. Anything that you take pride in can be a target rich environment for insecurities if you're not careful. Being prideful about your appearance, your body, or your expensive show car is not necessarily a bad thing if kept in perspective and in balance with the rest of your life. If, however, you place an inordinate amount of emotional weight behind how you look or the shininess of your chrome bumper, then develop a giant unicorn zit on your forehead or someone creases your side panel, your world will be off-axis and insecurities will emerge like ants in your cereal. So yes, I will give credit where credit is due. Depression forced me to discard my image, to show the world what I truly am, which is me. It would have preferred I keep it and killed myself, but I opted for the alternative.

So I picked up my trusty steed and headed out in search of the next box to check. The rhythm of days recently has been so different than what I have ever experienced. In years 1968 through 2019, there has been an understanding, a cadence to the day that gave it form and structure. I may not have liked what the agenda held for that particular day, but it was a known quantity. It felt real. Comparatively, the days recently have an element of the surreal, with riots and masks and Zooms. It feels like we're all living in an improvised reality show directed by Billy the Puppet, from *Saw*, that creepy little puppet-looking thing riding a tricycle.

I remember New Year's Day 2020 vividly, so many big plans, so much hope and optimism. "This is the Year of Rodger!" Losing my mom and suffering other setbacks in 2019, coupled with the symmetry of the numbers, how could 2020 be anything but a triumphant climax after a long, hard pent-up frustrating year? Through the first sixty days promise was ample, business was brisk, and the goals we fashioned into arrows were flying straight and true. Then some fucker in China at an undercooked bat. Everyone in the civilized damn world knows that you cook bat to an internal temperature of at least one hundred sixty-five degrees, and that it's best served on a mound of rice over a field of fresh greens sprinkled with a soy sauce and ginger reduction. How hard could it possibly be?

Before long, words and phrases once unknown, "COVID-19," "social distancing," and "flattening the curve," made their way across the Pacific faster than most Wish deliveries. Soon the unthinkable was being thought, businesses shut down, kids sent home to learn online, and we were told to shelter in place with no means of wiping our assholes. Overnight we had been classified as either "essential" or "nonessential" and treated accordingly. My "climax" of a year was quickly turning into a sandpaper dildo and any lube was being routed to those deemed more essential.

I was like most Americans in my level of unpreparedness. Overnight stores were emptied of food, alcohol, and, of course, paper of all form and function. Apparently Mad Max was all wrong. It's not going to be gas or water we fight each other for; it's going to be ass wipe. Lord Humungus, representing the ragtag post-apocalyptic tribe of Charmin will go on the loudspeaker, "There has been too much violence, too much pain, just walk away. Give me your three-ply, your baby wipes, and those paper towels that have more perforations that allow you to choose different sizes, and I'll spare your lives. Just walk away, and I'll give you safe passage to the human wastelands."

We began treating our neighbors like threats to our supplies. Never underestimate the speed that panic and mania can spread. It's like a wildfire, only way more dangerous. Ironic as it may seem, when there is real concern and genuine tension, my depression is fully in check. During times of crisis my darkness is nowhere to be found, not that I'm looking. Now I know the psychology and science of survival mindsets and how primary importance is put on survival and how the amygdala overrides normal frontal lobe functioning, but I don't buy it. My depression is cunning and devious. It knows better than to attack when I'm on highest of alert, so it waits in the shadows for the lull, for tensions to ease before springing its attack. The world is now sick, on the edge of pandemonium. Lisa found herself with a job but no work, Mack was fired from his job, Noah furloughed until further notice, and I was struggling to adapt to it all while preparing myself for imminent attack. Deep calming breath, focus on the inhale, focus on the exhale.

We don't play video games with adult diapers on, so we never have to push the pause button. We don't binge watch or purge watch anything, and I get bored with Netflix on the menu screen, so we lacked many of the modern skills that so many had been honing over the past few years for an occasion such as this. We made it through the lockdown by working out, by staying busy. We meditated and breathed, and I tried to stay vigilant as best I could by painting pictures or working puzzles, and then we would treat ourselves by putting on our best clothes and going to the grocery store to see if they carry imported crumpets and organic Swiss chevre, which apparently Walmart doesn't, so we'll try back tomorrow.

Then a man named George Floyd was killed, and the world descended into madness. Race has always been such a touchy subject in our country, and rightfully so, but until the mass protests spurred by Mr. Floyd's tragic and completely preventable death, I really had no idea how total and ingrained in our society racism truly is. Treating people different because of the color of their skin has always been a foreign concept to me. I know that is probably a "white" thing to say and would carry no meaning in the Black Lives Matter community, but if growing up in a town where I wasn't racist, where I didn't know anyone who was racist or encountered racism is privilege, then I am absolutely a child of privilege. In making a serious effort to hear what is being said by the Black community, I realize that I have been blind or unaware to racist historical backstories or context, and it has changed how I look at the world around me.

I will never apologize for who I was born, that is the apex of stupidity, but no one should have to live in fear because of who they are and shouldn't ever be treated differently because of the color of their skin or who they love. I feel sorrow for those whose lives are made challenging for nothing more than being born unique individuals and joy for those who rise above oppression with class and dignity and look forward to a time and place where all are treated equally and the only privilege is what is earned with time and effort. I personally feel that with a country as divided as ours, the only thing that will bridge the gaping chasm is to come together in joint hatred of something else, perhaps stupid tasty bats. In my opinion, in keeping with the unprecedented shit-showedness of 2020, I think at some point in the fourth quarter of this year earth will be attacked by a race of aliens from the outer reaches of the space whose only purpose is to enslave our dolphins and eat our paper, then we'll join hands across racial, political, and financial divides to shoot space freaks in the face.

Until the mother ship arrives, we'll do our part to stay safe and healthy, we will wear masks to help our community do the same and support those who are peacefully trying to equal the scales while steering clear of the assholes who just want to break shit. What we really need is the mother of all halftime speeches. We need a shot of adrenaline administered via long needle right through the chest to restore hope and get us excited that the second half of the year is ours to win. I remember my football days and the confidence I felt during pregame drills, envisioning what the victory would feel like, only to have our asses handed to us the first half. We sat in the locker room, dejected, wondering what the hell just happened, then the coach came barreling in, eyes red, ears smoking, and spittle flying from his yelling mouth. He told us that we're better than this, that we should expect more from ourselves and our teammates, then, still yelling, he walked over to the folding table with the jug of Gatorade and small waxed paper cups arranged neatly in symmetrical lines and, with a smooth, strong pull, flipped the table over. Amber liquid drops shimmered against the fluorescent lights and rained down upon us, and white cups littered the room. Coach was yelling, we were yelling, the game was back on, and we were still in it! With newfound vigor, we grabbed our helmets and headed back into battle. In the end we lost the game but looked better doing it, then headed to the locker room to clean up Gatorade and cups. That's what our country needs, just better and less messy.

It is unfortunate that in order for a halftime speech to be effective, you need believable leadership and faith and trust in your teammates, and both I feel are in short supply in this country at this moment in time. Personally, I don't care about who you vote for or what God you pray to. I'm unconcerned about the color of your skin or how much money you make. If you suffer from depression, I want you to know that you are not alone, times like these always have a way of making us feel even more isolated and distant from our fellow man. I want you to know that your life matters and what you choose to do with your life matters.

WEDNESDAY, JULY 8, 2020

It's been a while since I checked in with you to see how you are doing. It's always about me, me, me, I hope you're okay in your mind space, that you are eating right, exercising, getting sleep, and trying to be mindful and focused. I know some days you're the mower, and others you're the rock hit by the mower, becoming a projectile heading straight toward that plate-glass window. I don't know how to interpret that myself because I got shit sleep last night and feel mentally fettered right now. We use window air conditioners during the summer to keep us from spontaneously combusting, mostly because we have an old-ish house that was electrically wired by Clark Griswold, and last night that sombitch was complaining and vibrating. I wanted to yell "This. Is. Sleepy. Ni-night" and front-kick it through the window, but my leg doesn't reach that high anymore.

At some point as I'm taking the three walk-monkeys of the apocalypse around the block, I start feeling my generalized anxiety disorder kicking in. I haven't talked about my anxiety too much and its feeling a bit left out. You see, my anxiety was born not long after my apple tree depression mindfuck thing but has always been the runt of my psychotic litter. When something is trying to kill you, everything else ends up eating at the kid's table and wearing hand-me-down OshKosh B'Gosh. Not to say that my anxiety is a minor annoyance. What it lacks in intensity and terror, it more than makes up for in persistence and tenacity. It's constantly there like sand in your pubes after a day at the beach.

The big difference between my depression and my anxiety is that I gave birth to my anxiety, created and fashioned it myself, whereas my depression was implanted in my brain by a highly developed alien race conducting catch, probe, and release operations. Generalized anxiety disorder may have developed naturally for me, but I feel that there is a direct causal relationship between its growth and my depression. While I had a great childhood, it wasn't stress free. I had to go to church, where I learned about hell and how unless I became a way better a person than I was. All my mail would one day be forwarded there. School at that age wasn't about snacks and naps but about hormones, popularity, good hair, and learning facts and shit. I remember back to high school and college, remember basic training and my time in the Air Force. Stress was always a part of my life, often a significant part, but as hard as I try to pinpoint a time when that episodic stress turned to general anxiety, I haven't been able to nail that down.

Stress and anxiety are related but are not the same thing. Stress is a response to an external trigger such as an approaching deadline or getting caught staring at someone's breasts. Once that external trigger has passed or been resolved, the stress fades. Anxiety, on the other hand, is excessive and persistent worries that do not go away, even in the absence of any stressor. While my depression causes significant stress in my life from time to time, it cranks out worries like it gets paid by the bushel, six-foot, seven-foot, eight-foot jump off a cliff. Before I really knew it or had any concept of how to stop it, I had gained another constant unwanted companion that would forever be by my side.

It is amazing what a person is able to get used to. There is a lady named Ayanna Williams, who one day said "I'm not going to cut my fingernails ever again" and for over twenty years hasn't. She resides in the *Guinness Book of World Records* for longest fingernails at over nineteen feet long! Nineteen feet, you'd have to have your nails done at Maaco, and you could die picking your own nose. For Mrs. Williams, it's just another day, but could you imagine typing on a keyboard or sleeping or a truckload of other stuff that nineteen feet of fingernails would get in the way of for those of us not acclimated to so much keratin? Anxiety is far easier than that would be to become accustomed to, especially since we harbor a belief that we have earned our anxiety through our behavior or actions. We have done wrong or have not measured up in this world and in doing so have made the bed where we now lie.

I have begun to realize through my time in meditation and contemplation how responsible I am in creating and nurturing my anxiety. I have done so much in its creation. I have fed it, nurtured it, let it grow and prosper, that I should be able to claim it as a dependent on my taxes. I have become so comfortable with its existence that I no longer question its origin or veracity in my life. Here's an example. Every day I take the three tail-waggers for a walk we cover the same course, hang a right out of the driveway, followed by another two hundred fifty feet beyond. This leg is roughly two-tenths of a mile in length, and I use this time to let the dogs settle into their unsettledness. Once we hit the stop sign for our third right-hand turn, my mind shifts from replacing these damn neurotic dogs with turtles, to what the day looks like and what all needs to happen before the dinner bell rings. This is the spot where I cue my anxiety and a sick feeling starts to develop in my stomach. I tell myself that it's just the body experiencing coffee withdrawals, but I know it's not. It's a feeling as if I have forgotten something important, or have missed a call or email, and that someone is disappointed in me.

I have unwittingly created this "anxiety trap" for myself by trying to be efficient with my time management. My thought was that I would maximize my day by using all available brainpower during periods where it would usually be set to idle. It's like the old lawnmowers that had an icon of a rabbit and one of a turtle, and to get it to rev faster, you would rabbit that bitch up and get shit done. So when I would round that corner every day, when the dogs would expend enough energy to act like responsible pets and not like cracked-out gerbils, then I would take that time to plan and strategize becoming a captain of industry. I would do this every day, and it didn't take long before my thoughts would fixate on what I didn't do, leading to a morning recap of yesterday's shortcomings. Soon I had set an alarm for my anxiety, and each morning at the same time and place, the alarm would go off spurring another round of stomach-acid-inducing slow-motion play by play. That is exactly why the turtle beat the rabbit in the race. The turtle wasn't faster; the rabbit was just an asshole that went crazier than a fish with tits.

Once you live with anxiety about something, it opens the door to living with anxiety about everything, like inviting a gypsy into your home, or is that a vampire? My anxiety and depression have a symbiotic type of relationship, covering the same psychological territory but doing so in different ways. They are like a tag-team pro-wrestling duo that doesn't really fit together, like when Hulk Hogan teamed up with Mr. T on that one WrestleMania. My anxiety will set up my depression, will help it find a way in, will unlock the door to the castle if it knew where I kept it. It's in the cheesy plastic rock key saver thing under the mat by the way. My depression, on the other hand, doesn't lead to greater anxiety, preferring not to share the spotlight in the Neurosis Talent Show and Pie Raffle. Truth be told, I have always been so fixated on the depression that I have spent almost no time on dealing with the anxiety, as if I live on a sinking boat that's just a little bit on fire. I'm going to be throwing every ounce of energy at pumping out the bilges since it's just a small fire that statistically has a lower percentage chance of killing me than, say, drowning, because my boat sank.

One cool thing that I have learned about my anxiety lately is that it can be killed, "and if can be killed, we can kill it." I imagine Arnold Schwarzenegger saying that, wearing camo. What I mean is that individual anxieties specific to singular people, events, or circumstances can be singled out of the herd and shot in the face. This is one of the nifty things I have learned through meditation and contemplation. You see, my anxieties are just worries that I have done something wrong or in some unknown way created discomfort or disappointment in another being, by shedding light on that particular instance and following through with a series of questions such as "Is this anxiety justified?" and "What could I have done differently, if anything?" By just realizing that I did the best I could do in any one occurrence, or if I didn't, I gained valuable experience; it negates the value I have put on that particular anxiety.

The problem is that over the years I have buried these countless anxieties and promptly forgotten where, in essence creating a minefield for myself that I must walk through on a daily basis. Each step could unexpectantly set off an explosion of doubt and insecurity that could affect my day negatively. I have actually had anxiety about having anxiety, or anxiety squared. I haven't yet developed a plan or strategy that would work like a minesweeper rolling across my brain, so I'm dealing with individual neurosis as they present themselves. I will talk with Dr. K about it tomorrow at our session, which I am still looking forward to because of the outright progress that I've made. Maybe she could help devise something, or hypnotize me and say bibbidi-bobbidi-boo, so much of this brain stuff seems like magic or conjecture, but I find myself gaining an inkling of understanding as I work through it. It's like learning Spanish by watching telenovelas on Univision. *Amor* means "love," *comer el coco* means "to eat the coconut," and *mi carajo es grande* means "my dick is big."

I have learned a lot about myself and my anxieties over the past few weeks, especially when focusing on them and understanding the impetus that fueled their existence. I see know how my policy of moving forward at all costs prevented me from taking the time to process my feelings and validate the veracity of the circumstance creating the particular anxiety. I know that a common factor within the great majority of the anxieties I have been eliminating is my fear of disappointing people that, coupled with my other fear of exhibiting visible signs of depression or anxiety, in other words "not appearing normal," has created an environment where an assumption of deficiency exists. I guess what I'm trying to say is that every time I have a personal interaction where someone is not fully satisfied, whether or not I had any control over their satisfaction, it creates an unresolved anxiety. I will carry that anxiety into the very next interaction, which I assume will be another disappointment and so on.

I've been doing this shit for years. It's like saving your clipped toenails in a jar, for years. It's stupid and detrimental to your appearing like a normal human being. So goal number one going forward is not doing it again, which is going to be easier said than done. Like Ayanna Williams deciding to cut her fingernails, special tools will need to be acquired. I will have to bring a special mindfulness to all my personal interactions, paying special attention to the ones that may not have gone as planned. Maybe what I can do is keep a journal of sadness and disappointment where I write down how I felt I have let other people down, then go through it at the end of the day and contemplate each one. I don't want to make it sound like it happens every day or multiple times a day, just that when it does, it impacts me substantially. Again, therapy fodder for tomorrow.

I do believe that even with my current progress, I have given up hope on fully living a life without anxiety, which in itself is also a problem because without hope, there can be no belief, and I have to believe. For so long, my anxiety has been like a Rubik's Cube. The closer you are to getting all the green on one side, the more it fucks up the others, so more like a Rubixiety Cube. By the way, I named that; it's mine, and I'm going to patent it. I've had enough for the day. Needless to say, anxiety is a thing, and living with it sucks. I promise, from this day forward, to deal with it and prevent it from being an impairment to my future. The traps I have already set I will take care of in turn as they arise. That is all I can do, and I'm suddenly feeling okay with it, if not just a little more hopeful.

THURSDAY, JULY 9, 2020

I woke up after yet another restless night, tired, needing coffee and a full-frontal lobotomy. Thinking of the uphill climb that starts right now, I get up, make the bed, get some clothes on, and opt for AirPods and music, hoping it will keep me mellow and focused on my short-term goal of not ringing the breakfast bell for my anxiety around turn number three. I put the AirPods in the wrong ears, then the right ones, again wonder why they don't color code those bastards, get the three hopping Korean appetizers on their leads, and grab a poopy bag that I will use only if the offense doesn't go unnoticed. Somedays getting out the door with these three is the hardest part of the operation. It's like strapping on rollerblades and trying to escape a burning nightclub.

Like other morning, I let them burn off their excessive energy on the first leg of the journey, mindful of my target quickly coming into range. One hundred meters, ninety meters, eighty meters. I don't know why I'm using meters instead of feet. Are meters more dramatic? Regardless, I really don't have a plan other than to bring mindfulness to a part of my day that I had set to "automatic anxiety" hoping that would be enough to break the spell, at least for today. As I passed the spot without incident, I came to realize that I didn't need to light a candle or kill a chicken inside a cryptic symbol. Apparently, by the simple act of being aware of the trigger and by being mentally cognizant of not creating any new anxiety while breaking old anxiety cycles, I was successful in the attempt. I wouldn't say the rest of the walk was carefree. There is inherent stress when taking this pack anywhere, but today already seemed a bit brighter.

I'm sitting at the kitchen table, feeling buoyed by my early success, feeling pretty good about myself, except for my butt. I don't know why we don't have cushions on our seats. We used to. What happened to the cushions? Nevertheless, I bring my mind back to the present and what the day has planned, and it's going to be a big day, it's therapy day, and I already feel ghosts of old anxieties trying to tug me toward worry. Actually looking forward to a therapy session is a novel experience and goes far in putting those ghosts to their final rest. I need to work on ways to disassociate anxiety from basically everything that I do. It is only a fleeting sensation that I get, but I feel as if my depression is reeling a bit, that by systematically killing my anxiety, I am taking the fight to him and he is on his heels, looking for a counter. The mental image makes me smile. I really feel that for the first time I am allowing myself to get better, stronger, not giving in to the doubt of long-term efficacy or that I'm trying to drain the ocean with a leaking bucket.

I keep telling myself to do what I can if all else fails—get another cup of coffee, which I gleefully do. The act of rising to freshen my sadly empty mug is enough to push my anxiety away, at least for now. My sesh isn't until eleven, and I have a couple calls to make and emails to electronically mail, and my shirt isn't going to get wet all by itself. Having a healthy routine has absolutely saved my life during this smoldering exploded Hot Pocket of a year that has been playing out. It has kept me moving and proactive when all I really wanted to do at times was to grow my hair out and join a creepy traveling carnival where I would be in charge of the Tilt-a-Whirl or perhaps the Scrambler.

Five minutes early is right on time. Here I stand waiting for my appointment to begin, trying hard not to make eye contact with myself or check my nose hair, confident in the knowledge that Dr. K would choose that exact moment to enter the meeting. I have come to the conclusion that Zoom should have a knock feature on their waiting rooms that would give the participant waiting a moment to gather themselves or wake up, like in a real doctor's office. Suddenly, Dr. K arrives, right on time, and the therapy clock starts. We exchange pleasantries as civilized people do, then begin a quick recap of previous events before talking about the highlights of the past couple of weeks.

I realize as I relax into the moment and as the conversation evolves that something profound is occurring. Allowing myself, even through skepticism, for the briefest of moments to open up to something new like meditation without preconception of outcome, then experience success, has reset a paradigm somewhere between the folds of my brain. I no longer felt the compulsion to lie to Dr. K for the sake of expediency or to hold up an image of mental health. I even recounted to her some of my previous therapy experiences, especially my penchant for cutting corners and my preference for faux breakthroughs at the expense of real relief. A wry smile makes her face brighten as she says, "It happens all the time." Depressed people are habitual liars, not about regular stuff, not under oath or on their taxes, but certainly about their true feelings, about their depression and the deepness of their pain.

It felt good to "come clean," like I'm finally becoming a functioning adult, which I hope happens before I'm eligible for Social Security. I talk with Dr. K about the focus that meditation has been bringing me in a short amount of time and the realizations around my depression and anxiety. She nods approvingly, pleased with all that I'm saying, and I, in turn, am pleased with the genuineness of the words that are coming out of my mouth. For a moment I feel like I'm back in the fifth grade, giving my oral report to the class, and I'm fucking nailing it, the kids are enthralled, and I'm working the room, the teachers proudly smiling. During one of the brief moments I'm not talking, she looks at me and asks a rhetorical question but one that will serve as the basis for further discussion: "Do you think that being ready to do the work this time has made a difference?"

I, of course, know the answer but haven't really thought about it in that perspective. The words "ready to do the work" really pushed a button somewhere in my control room. I don't know what the button was for, but it started some gears moving, flywheels spinning, and sent stupid brain spiders scurrying. I am indeed "ready," readier than I have ever been before, but that isn't what is stupefying me at the moment; it is the realization that in my previous attempts

I wasn't. It takes a moment to sink in, forty years of dealing with this depression bullshit, different meds, different failed therapies, the comprehension that I was never ready to make a change, that skepticism and doubt has caused me to have a flawed approach and forsaken commitment to any treatment process. I can't help but let my mind imaging where I could be if I had been "ready" earlier. My first guess would be on a yacht anchored off the rocky coast of Santorini, playing cornhole on the teak quarter deck, soaking in the Mediterranean sun waiting for my helicopter with pontoon skids to land and take me to Starbucks.

I realize that this is the essence of flawed thinking. The fact that I am not ready is due in large part to the fact that I wasn't "ready," and while this may seem like the stupidest sentence ever written, it doesn't take away from the fact that it's undeniably accurate. I had not reached the level of necessity or desperation that would make me mentally willing and able to change. I know that there were times when I was at my lowest, ready to pay my bill and check out, that I had to be ready, just had to be, but on quick reflection, I realize that those times were about moving away from the pain and suffering, putting distance between me and my depression. Once that happened, I would resume my original course, until the next time.

I distinctly remember being admitted into the Johnson Unit at the downtown hospital. I know it sounds like what I call my penis, but in actuality it is a secure behavioral health ward affectionately nicknamed the Nut Hut by those temporarily residing within its walls. It is the place that depressed people go to "not die" when they are suicidal. Obviously by my very presence I was "ready" to make a change. I approached my stay in the Hut with an essential urgency, but I was less concerned about my life or issues as were the professionals treating me. There were no nuances or subtleties in treatment plan; it was more like "Why do you want to kill yourself, and how can we most expeditiously get you to not kill yourself?"

In honesty, I hated that fucking place almost immediately, and I hated myself for my weakness that put me there. The facility itself seemed comfortable enough, once admitted through a secure portal you find yourself in a large square room serving as a common area, appointed with matching chairs and benches made of stained wood and earth tone fabric. A nurses' station lived on the east side of the room, next to a hallway leading to the austere rooms containing little more than two wooden twin bed frames with a single plastic-covered mattress on each and two nondescript wooden shelves for personal items. On the north side was a small outdoor courtyard enclosed by twelve-foot-high solid fence and two potted Charlie Brown Christmas trees. The last room was my favorite, a large activity room with tables that reminded me of a high school science classroom used at various times throughout the day for diverse treatment options including art. There was more than an ample amount of beige, and while there was some amateur art displayed and a few token "hang in there" posters, there was blanker wall space than I would prefer.

For all intents and purposes, I was incarcerated, but like at one of those white-collar places where the gangs talk about feelings before shivving you with Water Piks. My fellow "inmates" were a core sample of the local society, ranging in income level and social strata from professionals to temporarily unhoused, and while it was a requirement to be "fucked up" for admittance, I quickly found out what a sliding scale that could be. For the most part, depressives stay to themselves, so you didn't have to worry about too much talking, except for the manics, when they were on a "high" you couldn't get them to shut up with a brick. My admission to this establishment arose from my wanting to kill myself, my desire to end it all, not from an attempt, and this stay was to provide a "circuit breaker" a time of respite and reflection that would move me away from the brink. After a couple of days, what I was most "ready" for was to get the hell out.

Check the men's room walls, and you'll quickly learn that I've been around, been around professionals of every kind, been around family and friends that have heard all the right words before. I couldn't come out all of a sudden "cured." This wasn't an old-timey revival meeting. I couldn't just all of a sudden say, "I was at my end, brothers and sisters, the devil had me by my short hairy nether regions, and he whispered into my ear, 'Do you know what he said dear congregation? He told me to kill myself by going out into the wilderness, loving people, to go out there and slather my naked body with Nutella and let a cougar maul my deliciously chocolatey hazelnutty flesh,' but I said, 'Devil, that's a stupid idea, and through the power of prayer I was saved, hallelujah.'" Then the doctors would stamp "cured" on a form and let me go. Nope, these docs have seen it all, have heard it all, and if I was going to talk my way out of this, it was going to have to be believable.

I hear you, believe me when I tell you that the irony is not lost on me, if I had just put the work in at this point instead of channeling energy to escaping the confines I found myself in. I would be much further along in my journey. In my stupid mind, the deception was providing me a mental challenge to overcome while still allowing the therapy to take hold and change my life. There were two individual sessions and one group session each day, with a sprinkling of activities, some required, others elective, throughout the day. I would go into the morning solo session and make sure that I said words like *thinking, working, feelings,* and *emotions,* making sure to remember what I said so I could expand on them later in the afternoon. The group therapy was fucking worthless, twenty people sitting in a circle wanting to be anywhere but sitting in a circle, not talking unless directly asked a question, except for the manics who loved the group environment because it was their time to shine.

I complained about taking meds and told them that they made me feel defenseless and want to kill myself. They nodded, wrote something down, and then made me take the pills they offered. I wanted to take them then hack my wrist open with the serrated plastic knife from the lunch tray just for spite, but since I was in "compliance" mode I took them with a smile and thumbs-up. Each day I would ramp up the story just a little bit in between naps, because fucking meds. Of course, you just can't keep getting better and better; it's not believable. You have to throw in a minor setback, like "antiquing" a piece of furniture with a few whacks or scratches. It makes it seem more believable. There was still clearly drama in my life waiting for me to get out, so I used that as an excuse to throw a fit, refusing to go to evening session or even eat dinner. I wasn't missing much since it was in point of fact, hospital food. Later that night, I overheard a nurse and an orderly talk about how good I was doing and thought "bingo."

The next day I came back strong, nailed the morning individual session, and began to think that this was "breakthrough day." I told the doc about how I'd deftly worked through the issues, how I was able to cope and handle random stressors now, and that I felt like a new man. I was told that the progress was a good start and that we'd see what tomorrow brings before making a decision, but you could feel the momentum starting to swing in my favor. I will say this about my stay at le hotel insanity. I was exposed to some pretty cool art therapy classes that would serve to rekindle my love of creativity and would be the longest-lasting positive impact of my time at the Johnson Unit. When I awoke the next day, I knew that this was it, one more session, maybe two, but just keep it up, and sure enough, later that morning, I was called into the administrator's office, where I was told that tomorrow morning I was being discharged.

I remember being excited that I had pulled it off, that the master plan had gone to, well, plan, but a nervous charge of electricity made my body shiver as I thought about what the hell I was going to do when the door opened. No question I was going quit the meds. For my own good, I was going to throw them in the first trash can I came across. Nobody worries about the side effects of suicide if you're on suicide watch and being constantly monitored, but on the streets, there is no time to be monitored. It's the law of the jungle, and you're either the lion or the gazelle, and neither of them take depression meds. As I finally was "buzzed out," breathing air outside the unit for the first time in weeks, I couldn't help but draw the correlation between my time within and those serving civil penalties in the jail across town for varying degrees of assholery. The focus is not on healing or rehabilitation; it is on gaining freedom from an uncomfortable environment, the moment that we are immersed into a forced compliance our primary objective is no longer in getting better but in getting out.

After what seems like hours, I snap back to Dr. K and our continuing session. She asks about my PTSD. I tell her about how this past Saturday had been the least anxiety ridden in months until it wasn't. I recount how a one second Josh outburst of vocalization had rocked my world, in the bad way. She is quiet, eyes down taking notes or drawing pictures of pirates or turtles. After what is almost an awkward passing of time, she looks up and asks, "What was most significant to you, the anxiety-free day or the intense PTSD episode?" I have to also wait a little longer than comfortable to formulate my answer since my gut reaction was to say "the PTSD" because of the impactful negativity and intensity, but then I have to think twice because it had been months since my Saturday hadn't been consumed by fear or worry.

Sensing my conflict, Dr. K reiterates something told to me the first time we met. "Your brain does not understand that at that moment it is not in immediate danger. It is telling you that it is being attacked or in imminent danger of attack, and these feelings are based on thoughts." She continues, "Let me reframe the question, did you find the PTSD most significant, understanding that it is based on thought, or the reality of having a stress-free Saturday." The answer hits me between the eyes, I choose reality of course, but it was a powerful example of the risks of an incomplete thought process, that there is usually far more to an issue just below the surface.

I take the moment of understanding to ask for more tools, more Jedi mind tricks to add to my growing arsenal and she explained to me that there is nothing more important than a willingness and pro-active nature. She encourages me to simply continue down the path that I had chosen, to grow in understanding before adding layers of complexity that may alter my course. I agree, of course, but still have a little twinge of disappointment, like when I had just gotten a toy but immediately wanted a new one, because it was new, but my parents would say, "No, go outside and make one out of wood."

Dr. K asks if I have come to any formal closure of my mom's passing, and I tell her that I haven't, but I think about her every day. My mother knew me as only a mom could. She knew my struggles maybe better than I knew them myself and wanted desperately for me to have the ability to quiet my thoughts and find a moments peace. She was calmed so much by water that she always wanted me to go sit beside a river and let it soothe me, and now upon reflection, maybe she was just telling me to go jump in a river. That may be an issue for another day, but the fact remained that she felt a spiritual calm and unity with God when she was near a murmuring brook or walking on the beach, with waves crashing at her feet. I'm not a praying guy, but I assume that it could be a lot like meditation, I know that in watching her it looked like she was meditating. She would read a passage in her Bible, then close her eyes and pray. In the weeks leading up to her death, she made me promise her that I would do as she asked, that I would find a peaceful stretch of moving water and just be. I haven't fulfilled that promise to her yet. I don't know why. I've been around rivers on several occasions. I could just pop down by the bank spend a little time, maybe throw a line in, but I haven't. Honestly, I've avoided it, for some reason I can't bring myself to do it, not yet anyway.

Somewhere in a room across town where Dr. K was sitting, a soft chime was heard, signaling the closing of this session. Before I knew it, and frankly before I was ready, our time together was over. With the improvements and progress that I had been making, a decision was made and agreed upon to continue down the path I had chosen, enhancing mindfulness and focusing on positivity and perseverance. The PTSD and anxiety firmly entangled with it would continue to be untied by my efforts, or it wouldn't. There was really no predicting something as erratic, but it was clear that good work was being done and that it should be earnestly continued. Our next session was already scheduled for two weeks from the day, so with that we exchanged friendly valedictions, and as fast as she appeared, she was gone.

I stood alone in Josh's room, staring at my reflection in the now blank computer screen, collecting my thoughts that seemed again to be spilling out of my ears and accumulating on the floor below. I walked down the hall, and like two weeks prior, Lisa offered the compulsory "How'd it go?" Once again, I looked at her and assured her that it was positive and that my brain is still processing, but that it was probably the most positive professional therapy appointment that I have ever had. She smiled a hopeful smile. She has been through so much of my depression psychosis traveling sideshow and non-amusement park roller coaster of absurdity bullshit that as much as I want contentment and stability for myself, I want to provide it for her even more. I am fully "ready" and have a newfound respect and understanding of what that means and the long journey it has taken me to get to this point.

I would say this if talking with a fellow sufferer, that nothing will fully and firmly take hold without the weight of genuine commitment behind it. For the best part of four decades, I have floundered aimlessly, like an actual flounder flapping around on a deck of a boat, wondering why both eyes are on one side of my face. If there is no readiness to change; there will be no change, at least not the long term, forever change that we all covet so dearly. That being said, how do you know if you're ready, and if not, how do you become "ready"? Truth be told, I didn't even know I was ready or not until it already happened. It's such a personal thing that only you will know the answer to, which is actually the way it should be since there is no greater expert on your depression than you, you've carried it, lived with it, perhaps almost even died with it, but don't make the same mistakes with yours that I have with mine. Find something and allow yourself the opportunity for that something to work. Don't allow skepticism or prejudice to impact your willingness to get some work done.

I realize now how big a part that my own stubbornness, wearing a costume to make it look like pride, played in my unreadiness, coupled with a "move forward at all costs" mentality that discounted or downplayed the importance of actually working through or successfully resolving an issue before it could grow into a neurosis. Like I said earlier, I regret nothing. I am the sum of my experiences, and if I had changed sooner, my whole space-time continuum would be fucked, and people in my photographs would start dissolving into obscurity. As it often happens, all of my setbacks and failures have set me up for my greatest success, which will be happening any day now.

FRIDAY, JULY 10, 2020

Do you know what would be the greatest? Getting a full night's sleep would be the greatest. A scene from the classic movie *The Sands of Iwo Jima* keeps flashing through my mind where John Wayne plays a Marine sergeant named Stryker, coincidently my next dog's name, who comes across a wounded soldier during a battle. As he reaches out to grab the tormented hero, the man locks eyes with Stryker and says "At least I'll get a good night sleep" before dying in an efficient military manner. My problem isn't getting to sleep and give me a pillow and five minutes, and I'll amaze your face. My problem is maintaining sleep. When I find my eyes open when they clearly shouldn't be, I don't get up, don't get a snack, or watch television or look at my tablet. I lay there and just try to not think, calming myself with the knowledge that my body needs rest just like my mind, and I don't want my body to be deprived of crucial rest because my mind is upstairs having zombie orgies at all hours. I have been having intense dreams, but I feel like this process is giving me insights and focus, helping me connect some of the subconscious dots that have escaped my understanding to this point. Of course, I could take a pill that would help me to sleep, and there's no shortage of options at the supermarket if I wanted to steer clear of pharmaceuticals as well, all-natural, organic options. Apparently I'm not the only one searching for a deeper relationship with Morpheus.

It's Friday, and that in and of itself used to be enough to make me feel good, especially during my drinking days, most especially if I had a drinky social thing later, and at some point I would end up feeling nothing but hungover the next morning. Outside inebriation and inside COVID-19, Friday is just another day to get up, make the bed, and take the shrunken mangies for a sniffing tour of the neighborhood.

I find myself feeling somewhat emotional and vulnerable this morning, even though I was able to block the arrival of anxiety once again at the usual predetermined meeting spot around corner number three. Therapy and healing open doors that you perhaps expected needed to be opened but didn't really want to open, like when you're a kid and hear strange noises coming from your parents' room, and you want to make sure that they aren't dying but also have this feeling like turning the knob would change your life forever. That kind of thing. Mind you, it's not like I have dark secrets that I want to keep hidden. There are no literal or figural skeletons hiding behind any of the doors of my conscious or subconscious mind. I never killed anyone or ran for public office or anything sketchy. You just want a degree of control over when certain doors open. Of course, you never have control, so when a door opens, you deal with it, but it sometimes leaves a rawness, a tenderness that leaves you feeling vulnerable for a period of time. I walked by the television, and at a glance I thought I saw David Hasselhoff, and I teared up momentarily remembering watching *Night Rider* with my family, knowing as an absolute certainty that one day my car would talk to me, that we'd be friends and banter, not this "low air" bullshit I've been dealing with for four months.

That is one thing that I found out about that I can caution those who follow in my footsteps. When you meditate and become mindful and open up all the wounds that had scabbed over, be ready; the feelings parade is getting ready to begin, and there will be happy floats and sad floats and balloons and Al Roker. It's all part of the gig apparently, but it has taken me by surprise how quickly I can shed a tear, how the stupidest things can suddenly have me wiping tears and snot off my face.

As I was on my computer dealing with an issue and getting ready for a big meeting I have later this morning, Lisa accepted a call from Nancy, and by the way her voice changed timbre, my heart sank as my mind formulated the assumption that Bill had passed. When

Lisa was finished, she hit the red button, sat the phone down, looked at me, and said, "David died." At that moment I was conflicted. My assumption was wrong. This is a failing common to assumptions. Bill was still with us on this mortal coil, which was a huge relief, but Lisa's cousin David, who lived in San Antonio, had unexpectedly passed away during the night. David and Lisa shared a unique intuitive bond that allowed them an immediate connection without the need for constant contact. David also had this unique ability to connect with Joshua on a level outside my understanding and would offer his insights to Lisa especially.

Two thousand twenty, the official year of the dick punch. My heart aches for Lisa, Nancy, and all of David's family and friends who have to walk through this new, fresh pain. As much as I want to call a time out, explain how this day has acted unfairly based on my hastily fashioned rules, and ask for an official do-over, the world, however, continues to spin on its axis, and soon I would be in an important managers meeting, so it was time to refocus my focus. I wanted desperately to attend the Zoom meeting in the "video off" mode knowing that my face was bearing signs of an emotional day, red eyes and viscous strands of snot randomly escaping my nostrils, but people want to see you, as well as hear you, making sure that you're not playing poker or flipping crepes. I put on a collared shirt, took off my *Land of the Lost* Sleestak hat and, just like that, became business Zoom compliant, five minutes early, right on time.

While I find my job very rewarding, at times it can also run the spectrum between utterly amazing to downright terrifying, the one thing that it has a multitude of is oversight. Everything that I do is seen, reviewed, and scrutinized, and any inaccuracy or mistake is immediately brought to my attention, by no less than one person. Sometimes more, but no less than one. Goddamn TPS reports. Today's meeting is with my "home office manager," for lack of a better term, even though she lives halfway across the country from the home office, but hell according to my Zoom background, I live in Castle Grayskull with my sister and cat, and roam Eternia protecting the people who reside there from evil Skeletor.

I don't want to be in this meeting, not even a little bit. I am not ready emotionally or mentally for a business meeting, but there is a lot of ground to cover, so I keep it together and dive in. Like many humans I imagine, I'm good at some things and less than good at others. I can work with a client, create rapport, build trust, and help them walk through a difficult decision-making process. I am far less capable of keeping track of all the books and records and procedures and operational systems, and I can fuck up an email faster than you could say, "Hey, you fucked up this email."

By the time this meeting was over, it clocked in at just over two hours, breaking my previous long Zoom meeting by almost thirty full minutes. I have been in longer meetings, but those were group affairs with lots of people, making it far easier to stop my video and flip some freaking crepes. I have found myself feeling less and less connected with people the more I have to use technology to connect to people. It's not just a feeling of disconnection, it is a feeling of anger and frustration coupled with a strange disenchantment like self-schadenfreude, which I just made up and now own. The fragile emotionality I have experiencing today has not changed, except for the worse. It has been a grind since far earlier than I would like. I have to do a far better job at doing the stuff I don't want to do in my life, which just may be the title of this book, that or *Flying Monkeys and the Art of Living with the Perfectly Sized Penis*. Like you, I wish I was more amused by this, but I'm still feeling crestfallen and inadequate, not about the penis thing but just in general. I'm going to invoke the twenty-four-hour rule and move on.

Oh, you don't know about the twenty-four-hour rule? Well, let me enlighten you. When something bad happens or I'm having a bad day and no matter how much I pull up, I'm still barreling toward a fiery impact with a mountain I will invoke the twenty-four-hour rule and allow myself some time to just wallow in doubt and self-pity. I can throw a hissy fit, be a whiny little bitch, and shake my fist at God, yelling "Why me!" At the end of the period, I simply move on normally like it never happened. I feel like I've validated my feelings without giving in to them and without originating a long-term negative cycle. The same thing is true about the rare occasions when I win or experience achievement. I get one day to feel like total hot shit, send God a high five yelling "I'm master of the freaking universe!" and basically act like a douchebag, without the long-term effects of actually becoming a douchebag. The twenty-four-hour rule allows me all the feels, which is good, without promoting long-term emotional trends. Knowing that there is a finite end to the good or the bad opens up the feelings without a complex explanation process. Just do your time and move on.

This rule, like so much else that I have created in my life to create ease and attain normalcy, has a bad side, an unforeseen consequence. Whenever anything is micromanaged there is the tendency to not fully explore all possible outcomes or to not closely monitor all elements and how they interact once introduced with each other. What? You not smelling what I'm selling? Oh, you just think at this point I'm just thesaurus-ing a bunch of random words together? Okay, let me give you an example. In the southern part of our state lies a large lake and small city where many of our amazing clients live and require service and meetings. The lake covers a significant area, and much of it is calm and shallow promoting a thriving mosquito population. Now since mosquitos are vile communist suck-monkeys and serve no purpose on earth other than to torment taxpaying citizens with bites that you can't not itch, especially if you think about them, then they get worse and you just want to cut your forearm off. Mosquitos had to go, so bring in the micromanagers.

The powers that be came up with the bright idea of bringing in a species of tiny bugs called midges that would eat all the mosquito larvae, which is gross, but would dramatically reduce the mosquito population. It was a plan that probably looked good on paper, with cartoon drawings of bugs eating baby bugs, and on the surface, it worked a treat; mosquito populations plummeted. This is the unforeseen part. Midges loved the area so much that their population exploded beyond control or reason, so when you drive around the lake you will hit walls of midges that make your windshield look like a small insect reenactment of the battle of Gettysburg, only with less horses and more splattered guts. Now midges are becoming a problem, so they will look at bringing in frogs to manage the midges, then cobras to manage the frogs, then tigers to manage the cobras, then armed redneck "patriot" militias who will manage the tigers with posturing and rhetoric.

Not to boggle minds but you just can't make a change within a system without said change creating a "ripple" effect that echoes throughout eternity. Now bringing it back to my twenty-four-hour rule, which was developed as a stop-gap measure preventing a bad day from becoming a bad week and so on. What I unwittingly did was to strengthen and solidify the "just push it down and move forward at all costs" mindset that I had, which at that point wasn't a negative consequence. Now, however, that's turned bad, like "Hollywood Hulk Hogan" goddamn Hollywood influence. Now my life is not about burying but of illuminating and how does that fit in with my twenty-four-hour thing? The answer is clear and simple—it doesn't work, not at all. I'm going to have to come up with a system that works within the plan, or revoke the twenty-four-hour rule altogether, shit.

I have to hold the working through of issues inviolate. This is how I will move forward without carrying forward. What that means is that, for now, I have to deal with my raw moods, my depression-induced psychosis, my bad days as they come, which sucks for time management, because instead of just grabbing a cup of sweet nectar of life with a little cream and writing the day off, I have to categorically deal with David's passing, process Bill's cancer, and deal with work stresses, all while having the emotional stability of a fifteen-year-old girl during prom season. Okay, there is nothing that I could have done about David. I can send flowers, thoughts, and prayer, but there is little else I can offer from across the country, so I feel a sense of conclusion, at least for this day. As far as my general grumpiness and somewhat caustic outlook for the day, there are several aspects at play. First off, I've been sleeping like a death row inmate with a circle on the calendar, which I feel plays a big role. Not having the easy out of drinking myself to oblivion could be playing a bit-part, though my missing of those foolish nights and queasy mornings is decreasing steadily over time. I can't also disregard my generalized feelings of impending doom that this year has injected into all our lives.

Upon reflection I have come up with the conclusion that there is no one reason for my uppity-ness. I simply have a burning corn cob up my ass. I'm manstrating or perhaps just caught a case of crankxious frown syndrome. What I have to become aware of is that a bad mood doesn't have to be related to depression and anxiety; it doesn't have to have a deeper meaning or have more to it than just being human on a particular day when that is far less easy than it seems it should be.

Hear ye! Hear ye! The twenty-four-hour rule that has been a standard operating procedure for many, many years has, from this moment forward, been revoked. In its place will be the exploration and processing of issues relating to or emerging from but not limited to depression, anxiety, ill-temperament, and all forms of chronic douchebaggery. I'm, like, 80 percent sure this is the right way to go. Making changes isn't going to always, or ever, be easy, but this feels like it jives with my overall direction, away from "Forward at all costs" toward "Forward, when it won't cost me future anxiety or pain." I know, that tagline sucks, but it, like me, is a work in progress. I have yet to fully understand how this will play out with future bouts of depression or future successes, but I'm looking forward to finding out.

When I was a kid Saturdays were TITS, I lived for them, I would sleep in until eight, wake up, grab my pillow and comforter off my still warm bed, and head downstairs where I would plop down on the living room floor in front of the massive half-ton television set, and turn on cartoons. While the old cathodes and diodes warmed up, which could take several minutes before sufficiently ready to show a colored picture on the screen, I went into the kitchen and grabbed a plastic mixing bowl. For what I was about to endeavor one of those fake porcelain "bowls" was far to petite and lacked satisfactory capacity. This was no time for an amateur bowl best suited for something with a Gerber label on it, for it was cereal time and I was headed to the pantry, where I would put equal parts of each representative cereal in to my mixing bowl and then mix them with milk and sugar to the greedy top. I sipped the milk from the bowl as I made my way to the warm glow and tiny sound of the only television set in the house, where I had dibs, since I had staked my claim with ruffled bedclothes. I was master of the RCA. Of course, around this time, my parents, brother, and sister were stirring, but they were going to have to watch *The Batman/Superman Hour*, then Looney Tunes before finishing up the morning with *Hong Kong Phooey*, whether they liked it or not.

So much has changed in the almost forty years since that it makes me sad. I can't tell you when the last time I slept until eight was, cereal is now the Dark Lord Carb-Mor who must be eschewed, not chewed, sugar will kill you until you die from it, and today's cartoons are as unimaginative and irrelevant as their target audience.

Up until last week my recent Saturdays were only slightly different, I would wake up, work out, get coffee, start to have anxiety about the upcoming visit from Josh, and worry about something breaking down, besides me, that is, and look forward to getting through the day. Last week a good deal of the same stuff happened except for the excessive worry about Josh, which buoyed my spirits and restored my hope in achieving a degree of normalcy at some point. This week is, for intents and purposes, largely identical, but then again it isn't. You see, today is Big J's haircut day, which is its own thing. Josh hates haircut day and has broken more shit and caused more blood to flow on haircut day than at any other time, except maybe nail-trimming day. It's not that I'm super nervous, but it's a bit like being a plump delicious chicken, and Josh is a tiger coming for a visit. He looks well fed but there's this glimmer in his eye, and then you whip out the clippers, and that glimmer turns into rage, and then you can imagine the rest.

Lisa has always cut Big J's hair, from his first to today. She's done the clipping and paid the highest price. When things were really bad, I would offer my body up as a buffer between him and hers hoping beating on me for a time would slake his bloodlust. Behavior medications have gone far in the amount and severity of violence that presents itself on haircut day, but there are always signs of scratching and pinching on Lisa's hands and forearms when she is done. I have been told my management, Lisa, that I am to vacate the premises while she performs the delicate operation. The reason for this is mainly because I get very nervous when the clipper turns on and probably more so since my PTSD situation, and since Josh is highly intuitive, he picks up on that negative energy like microwaved Indian food in the break-room. So I will go to the coffee shop and not add any negativity to a tense situation, and Lisa will text me the "all clear" if she still has fingers and a phone when it's over.

I take my computer and Noah and get set up at my favorite coffee place. The coffee is dark and hot and soothes me, but my thoughts are not far from Josh and Lisa doing their not-happy dance at home. I remember the first *Playboy* magazine I'd ever seen was at my first barbershop. It was sitting in plain view on the coffee table next to a *Sports Illustrated* in between two rows of brown Naugahyde chairs with curved chromium metal legs shaped like a squashed letter S that lined the long walls of the rectangular room. I was with my father, in the company of other men of varying ages and hair account balances patiently waiting for their chance to take a withdrawal. I desperately wanted to pick up the magazine and thumb through it to see the holy grail of pubescent erotica, the nipple, but fear of God striking me dead or blind for engaging in fornication of the eyes had me reaching for the sports magazine to read about stupid nipple-less Wayne Gretzky. It was probably for the best, given the loose-fitting midthigh shorts that I would often wear in those days. This was my first glimpse at what is called an "old boys' club," grown men, smoking cigarettes, cigars, and pipes. The only thing missing was a brisket, talking sports, politics, and women, nonliteral jovial dick measuring. It was engaging and disgusting at the same time.

I remember the barber's name, it was Wayne, but I would call him Playboy Wayne, not out loud so my mom could hear, because if she found out I was going to a den of iniquity, it would be the last time I would be so close to not seeing anything. Haircuts have always relaxed me, except for the times Lisa wanted to cut my hair outside in the summer and the clipped strands would stick to the sweat on my warm body making me look like a Sasquatch with alopecia. Wayne preferred adult conversation, and since talking about boobs was far more intriguing than *Thundercats*, just sitting there was the extent of my responsibilities. The most enjoyable part was the straight razor shave, which for me was mostly ceremonial, and the hand massage that would immediately follow. I remember he would put this chrome box on the back of his hand with a toggle switch that, once activated, gave his hand magical properties.

Josh doesn't give a shit about the "experience." My guess is that a *Playboy* would end up in tiny little flesh-colored scraps outside his bathroom window, and having a straight razor anywhere near him seems like a criminally stupid thing to do. The only thing he hates more than a haircut is taking too long for a haircut. As soon as Josh sits down, Lisa is on the clock. It's like cutting the hair of an activated bomb, with a timer counting down, but also doing a good job, because Lisa has exacting standards and won't accept a less than standard haircut, even if she has to take a beating. If J explodes, Lisa will let him vent and hit the most expensive thing in his vicinity, before calmly asking him if he's ready to finish. A haircut may take several of these such outbursts before she is satisfied that he is "outdoor world" ready.

My part of this operation is going smoothly and that makes me feel guilty, like my platoon was called into action on some foreign shore, and I was left behind to apparently drink coffee, which honestly is my strongest game. I have to fight from thinking about what could be happening just three point two miles away. Images of Josh running through the house screaming, trying to rip out whatever plumbing he could find, holding a toilet plunger for some reason, with a screaming Lisa right behind him flood my mind—I have to actively force them away. Guilt is fertile ground for my depression, and it will use it masterfully against me, so I need to be fully on guard, and since the self-imposed moratorium on just burying shit, I need to fully work through my issues and not give it any kind of foothold. This one is actually pretty easy, given my recent episodes of PTSD, there would be an almost 100 percent chance of a recurrence if I had stayed at home, and since I play no real active role, there was no reason to be exposed to the potential. Even though I fully understand the thought process, which will alleviate any anxiety associated, I still feel the pull toward feeling like I should be doing more, or in some way that I'm deficient in my duties. I tell myself that I've put years in, gone through things most people can't imagine, that it's all right to sit a few plays out. For some reason knowing that I have done far more for my family than any random "deadbeat" dad comforts me.

If anyone were to ask what I hold dearest, what I'm most proud of in this life, I would say being a father. Because of the priority and seriousness that I put into that role, every aspect has a heightened degree of significance. That means when I fail, I fail big; when I feel guilt, I supersize it. With Josh and Noah both being autistic and requiring special consideration, the possibility of failure and feelings of inadequacy are even greater. I have always felt that my role as father is to help make my children's lives better and especially in the case of Josh that I haven't been able to accomplish that task. Now I'm aware that his autism is not due to me masturbating to the Sears lingerie catalog when I was fourteen or because I tried chewing tobacco in high school. I know Josh's condition was in no way caused by an action of mine or as a punishment from God, but I have this huge box of guilt and guilt-related neurosis upstairs that has Josh's name on it that I will have to deal with at some point.

I feel that I have given this moment in time sufficient respect and weight and that there is no reason to wallow in an unjustified feeling. I will put off opening that Josh guilt box until a time when I have the desire and mental resources to fully handle the process, but I won't be adding more to it today, which is positive and significant. I'm getting used to the "work through it" thing. I've come to realize in my advanced age that most "normal" guilt requires your permission before it can affect you, meaning that you have to be an active participant in its creation and nurturing. I have this whole "thing" about depression and guilt that I have been preparing for you, complete with interpretive dance and fireworks, but that's going to have to wait, because I just got a text from Lisa. It seems that the operation is complete, and it is now safe for me and Noah to return home, so I pack up my stuff, down the last lukewarm swig of coffee, don my plague mask, and head toward the door.

I walked into a calm environment with no outward signs of violence or disturbance, the quiet was eerily disturbing. I found Lisa folding clothes in the laundry room and asked for a recap of events. She told me that, all things considered, it went as well as could be expected. Holding up her hands to display the backside, a couple spots of red, irritated skin could be seen where Josh pinched her but altogether not a bad outcome. Let me take a minute to talk about being pinched by Big Man J. Most people have been pinched in their life, for most it was early, like on a playground in elementary school when that was a legit weapon, like the Indian burn, which was not named by me, I'm just perpetrating the, no, that's not what I meant, I was just a child and, well, shit. Pinches don't have to be weaponized, who doesn't like a playful yet appropriately respectful booty pinch from time to time? And unless you've hung a crawdad off your nipple, could you even call yourself a redneck? Well, you haven't been pinched in earnest until you've been pinched by my boy, he takes it to the next level. One of the few times Josh will lock eyes with you is when he pinches and grips your skin between his strong thumb and pointer fingers. He wants to see the look on your face as he moves his fingers back and forth, pushing constantly deeper, as he flexes his fingers, digging his fingernails deep into your skin, often drawing blood. Once he pinched the soft fleshy underarm area so hard, I screamed like a little girl and had a black bruise the size of a bottle cap, only bigger.

Lisa's wounds showed a lack of commitment on Josh's part in the inflicting of pain category, which is a good thing. I don't wasn't to diminish what Lisa went through. We've both been through so much worse, and she would just shrug it off anyway since that's her baby boy. I checked on the big man, and he was lying naked on his bed watching a movie, eating a Pop-Tart. Soon he would be getting in the shower and heading back to his house. Some positive things happened today that I don't want to overlook or take for granted. Where once I would have experienced a highly stressful day, complete with an episode of PTSD, today, for a haircut day, was about as stress-free, for me, as I have ever experienced. Now I know that was because I wasn't present for the hard part, but that, in and of itself, is also a step in the right direction, and doing it without inviting my depression for a long visit or adding to my large vault-o-guilt was a win-win.

Do you ever feel like life is just moving from struggle to struggle, trudging through mud, looking up a steep vertical path fraught with peril? That each new day brings you no closer to your goal? You are not alone, believe me. I feel you all over, not literally, because that would require explaining. Here's what I will tell you—small wins and tenacity will win the day…eventually. A mindset of not stopping no-fucking-matter-what, coupled with small goals and small wins is critical. Life will get easier, not because life ever gets easier but because you get stronger, and I know what you're saying—slap that shit on a picture of a newly hatched baby turtle struggling to get to the ocean and hang it up in the breakroom next to the vending machine. I'm hoping that because I said it, there will be a transformation from cheesy motivation fodder to genuine experiential wisdom passed from master to padawan, not that I'm a master or you're a novice, just that, um, shit.

SUNDAY, JULY 12, 2020

While Sunday isn't my favorite, I'm pretty sure I bitched about it earlier. I do like the option I have given myself of "sleeping in" one day a week until the sun's at full strength or six thirty, whichever is earliest. That extra hour and some just feels luxurious, like I'm moved on up to the east side, where the fish don't fry in the kitchen and beans don't burn on the grill, you know, like a "deluxe apartment in the sky" type of thing. I don't know why that just popped into my head, but I'm going to go with it. As soon as my feet hit the floor, I'm down the hall, opening the door so the dogs can do their business, and I'm pushing the "brew" button on the coffee maker. We used to have a fancy coffee maker that you could program to start at a certain time, but like everything else with a computer chip or circuit board, as soon as it senses your reliance on its operation, it goes "tits up," leaving you coffee-less and without defense when Skynet will one day launch its offensive. So in prepping for the apocalypse, we went with the cheapest, least computery model of coffee maker available on the market, which means I have to walk down the hall and push a button every day, which is my way of fighting back against the machine overlords.

It is a beautiful morning, clear blue sky, warm rays descending from the heavens as birds sing a melodious, calming chorus of chirps and tweets, until the fucking crows start in with their callous incessant ca-caws, that make you long for the days when you kept your trusty BB gun close at hand. Despite the murderous crows, I revel in the picture perfection of this time and vow to make the most of this bright summer morning. After the non-artificially intelligent coffee maker had given its all, and all that remained was a dark brown stain on the bottom of the carafe, I decided that a walk was in order, so I asked Noah if he wanted to join me on a stroll and being the awesome person he is, nodded, and went to grab his hat and sunglasses.

We walk down the street, it's still early enough on a Sunday that traffic, both car and pedestrian, is light. Where the street intersects with another, we cross over and head toward a bike bridge that will allow us passage over the freeway and to the "natural area" that is on the other side. Noah is a man of few words, so when we walk together, I am able to center my thoughts and be more mindful as I walk, which feels a lot like progress. Our walk covers about two and a half miles and allowed us the opportunity to enjoy some cool flowers and some different species of birds, one was small and plump looking, and one had red spots on its head.

My father seemingly knew everything. When asked what kind of bird that was, he would reply, "Oh, that's an *Ardea herodias*, or great blue heron, found throughout the temperate continental region, especially near water." When queried about that interesting flower, he would say, in a tone implying that the question was far beneath his ability to answer it, "Well, son, that's what we call a tricolor monkeyflower, which grows seasonally in wetter environments." I thought he pulled half his answers straight from his ass, but after a brief fact check, he was right; that was a goddamn tricolor monkeyflower. My dad was so cool and knew so much, but how? How do you get to a place where you know everything, when you're the one with all the answers, the simple ones and the hard ones? Like why do some people have brains that want to kill them, or why does feeling alone hurt physically?

I began to subconsciously want to know everything, to be the go-to guy. I don't think it's uncommon for sons to want to grow up to be their fathers, and I had one of the best. I started by reading the first volume of these encyclopedias that Lisa and I stupidly bought when I was in the Air Force, thinking that they would give our family a leg up on everyone else who would have to go to a library to learn shit. They weren't even from *Britannica*, they were American, probably printed in China. Regardless, I think I got through aardvark before thinking two things: one, the aardvark is a unique and mis-understood creature, and two, this was a stupid fucking idea. But as it turned out, it wasn't the stupidest fucking idea. That was my next avenue, which was reading the dictionary, figuring that every word written in every book is contained within one text, and by studying it, you would by proxy be studying everything. I know now that was flawed thinking, but I hungered to know everything. I just didn't know how to learn everything, and yes, I get the irony.

The pressure that I put on myself to be more like someone else had a real negative impact on my life and gave my depression an erection. It now had another chink in my armor for which it, and its good buddy anxiety, could exploit, which they did, early and often. This little cabaret was totally self-inflicted as I piled pressure on myself to be more, while life was putting regular pressures upon my shoulders, then there was the societal pressures and family pres-sures all heaped together to a point where your knees buckle, and you feel like you haven't lived up to anyone's expectation, and oh, the inglorious disappointment. For my depression, this was like walking into Costco a half hour before closing and having the once stingy sample givers offer you, however, many goat cheese hazelnut balls or gourmet squirrel meat savory tarts you can handle, since they have to clean up before quitting time. This was a rough patch for me, finding myself farther down the rabbit hole that I ever wanted to be.

In the end, I crawled out, slowly, methodically, one f-ing day at a time, and in so doing learned that I am not my father but also that I didn't have to be my father. That was one of my first early break-throughs. That victory not only took tremendous pressure off me but got me out of wearing a tie every day. When you're in the mud and muck, crawling and grasping for every inch, self-image takes on a whole different perspective. You see yourself differently, you see your situation differently. I emerged truer to what I felt I was, not what I wanted people to think that I was. I wasn't a fancy-car-driving, silk-tie-wearing, know-everything, put-together person. I was a scared, depressed, unsure but real person, and that was a start. So many peo-ple struggle to reinvent themselves day after day, and I know from experience how exhausting that can be.

I've had a couple of epiphanies lately thanks to the opportunities provided by COVID-19, the year 2020 and the letters F and U. First is that I feel that there has been a huge resurgence in the importance of image, that will have negative consequences in the near future. More and more people are putting emphasis on material things, new car sales are up and buying "toys" like boats and campers and chainsaw dildos are at an all-time high. That coupled with an unprecedented ability to redefine who we are and represent by simply pressing a button and changing our background from where we live, to where we want others to think we live. I've been on Zooms with powerful people in the Oval Office, with rich people in their high-rise apartments overlooking central park, with super-creepy people with their bondage chains and leather whips, and as I say that, I begin to realize that might not have been a digital background. The problem is that by constantly immersing yourself in that virtual image, that it will at some point conflict with your personal self-image and cause some disproportion in your operating system. I may be wrong, I have been before, but I am also no stranger to this ground and how easy it is to become overcome by inequities in how you see yourself.

I don't know if the first one was a true epiphany or was just a deep thought, which happens so rarely that I want to increase its significance to a greater lever. This one I firmly feel satisfies all epiphany requirements, which you could probably look up, in an encyclopedia. Humans are wired for connection with other humans, with our environment, our livelihood, our individual world. I have gone through periods of missed connection on many occasions before coronavirus was a thing. Many people who are actively going through depression have experienced the same, withdrawing from human contact, not venturing outside the narrow confines of the "golden triangle" couch to bathroom to bedroom, and basically hoping the earth would break free of its orbit and be left spinning through the galaxy like a cosmic game of dodgeball. Each time I was out of touch and regained my stability, I realized how much I missed and needed those connections. When boredom and mania took over recently, I decided to complete a thousand-piece puzzle, for time. I completely failed since every damn piece is the same damn color, but the attempt got me thinking about each individual piece and its unique shape. I began to see every piece and its distinctive loops and sockets, tabs, and slots as people who mesh perfectly with their surroundings just the way they are made. If I or someone else tries to change those characteristics to match a preconceived idea of how we should be shaped, not only will all connections feel forced and fake, the picture will forever be out of focus.

So when someone asks me what kind of tree that is, I will confidently answer, "It's a green tree, they grow all around here." Being true to yourself is liberating but is also a big responsibility because you begin to realize the obligation owed to yourself to be your best version. It means honestly owning your good, bad, and ugly and having real conversations about your depression and how it affects you at any given time. And since life is a long game, hopefully, it means constant diligence as who you are evolves over time. Something of the conversation I had with Dr. K bounces around my brain cavity as we round the corner of our driveway and head toward the door, and that was the importance of self-compassion.

I put a bookmark in my thoughts to be revisited later and got to work on my list of Sunday chores. Lisa and I decide to take our bikes out, and there's a great path about thirty miles down the road that runs along a river and around the side of a lake, so we load up the truck and hit the road. Today, life is easy. I'm not plagued or beleaguered by my depression or anxiety. They are taking the day off, which in a way is disheartening, thinking they are together in a "war room" with a tabletop battlefield overlay of my brain, and they are pushing little tanks and planes around with long sticks with flat wooden blades on the end. I push the worry aside, figuring I'll fight that fight when it rings the front door and lock the truck door as we don our helmets and mount the bikes. The first couple of miles follow gentle sloping farmland lined with trees and quaint houses, and horses and cows far outnumber cars and people, instilling a sense of peace. A few bright white clouds contrast the deep blue sky and overall provide a perfect environment to allow my mind of leash to wander around, somehow finding its way back to the idea of self-compassion.

Honestly, if I were a guest in my own mind and was writing a Yelp review based on my visit, I would only give it one star and leave a snarky comment: "This establishment has no idea how to run a brain. I would rather stay at Gary Busey's mind or even, dare I say, Weird Al's." It's not just the depression, not just the anxiety. It's the constant pressure that I put on myself and lack of understanding or compassion I show myself when I fall short. I feel that I have almost unlimited compassion for animals, for some people, not all but some, even insects get some measure of compassion. Not spiders, spiders can go fuck themselves. I reserve very little compassion for myself, opting instead for the highly effective option of berating, nit-picking, and holding myself to impossible ideal, just so I can say "I told myself so." If that doesn't make sense, then you're probably "normal."

As we round the corner and catch the first glimpse of the lake, I ponder how much easier my life could have been if I had cut myself some slack every once in a while. This is a passing thought, not a regret, because it would be the same as regretting not taking my private jet to Fantasy Island for afternoon tea with Mr. Rourke, where we would sit on the veranda and be served by Tattoo, and I would pat his head even though I knew it was inappropriate. In order for a regret to be deemed "legit" it has to actually be based in reality, and I had no concept that self-compassion was actually a thing. In my mind failure is weakness, even if I have set myself up for that failure by requiring more than I could give, it was not something to be accommodated, taken lightly; it required rebuking and stern discipline. As I look through my past with wiser eyes, I realize how I have played into my depression, how I have given it power. I believed that I had to be stronger, tougher than it to survive, but in that belief, I ended up breaking myself down, playing right into its hands, actually making it easier for it to negatively affect me. Stupid, see, that's exactly what I'm talking about.

If you, like me, were wondering what it is and how it works, let me through the divine power of Google enlighten you. Self-compassion is simply offering kindness to yourself at times of perceived inadequacy or failure. So when I shit the diet bed and eat a whole box of Little Debbie's Peanut Butter Crème Sandwiches, instead of running and putting on my plastic "sauna suit" while berating myself as a weak-minded, worthless, fish-lipped, grease-licking, tree-species-not-knowing, aardvark-appreciating loser, I should tell myself that I am only human, that Little Debbie is a vile temptress and that while it's okay to fill an apparent "hole" with peanut butter crème, that healthier options are available that will feed both body and soul.

We pull into an alcove at lakes end that has weathered picnic table overlooking the shimmering water and heavily wooded hills beyond and decide to take a minute and be present before starting the ride back. I think about self-compassion, still trying to wrap my head fully around the concept. I guess my biggest hurdle to overcome is my fear that I will "lose my edge" by being too easy on myself, that I will compassion myself into soft flaccidity, and that it will set me up for catastrophic failure in the future. We've all had assholes in our lives that "take a mile" constantly when offered an inch or can't get their act together at our expense, that we are forever covering or making excuses for and I don't want to be that person for myself, and for sure not for someone else. So while I do feel that there is room in my toolbox for self-compassion, I can see using it sparingly at first until I actually comprehend how it will impact me and provide benefit without giving up control.

And there it is, the dreaded C-word; I said it. I realize that as a rule I not only expect myself to live up to ridiculous standards, but to do so handicapped by obstacles that I throw in my path, knowing that failure will bring reprimand and retribution. If your question to me would be "Why would you do such a thing to yourself?" the answer is brilliant in its simplicity and stupidity—it's all about control. I get being in the "comfort zone" of discomfort with my depression and anxiety. I know the dark. I live in the dark and while it sucks donkey, to me it's a tangible "known." I can navigate and function and survive, whereas when I experience elation, optimism, or general "winning," my mind doesn't quite "feel right." It's like when you spend the day on a boat and reach shore but still feel the swells. I guess I feel exposed and vulnerable when I'm on a "high" and that by injecting kindness into the equation, I am facing a loss of control. I know that it's hard to understand, even for me, but it really is like becoming institutionalized, where your reality is built around a strict set of harsh circumstances that you almost come to expect and require to such a degree that "freedom" is a scary prospect.

That being said, I can't keep a smile from creasing my face as we make it back to the truck. I feel contentment and satisfaction, and in this moment, I could absolutely see the benefit of self-compassion, especially if it would allow more moments like this, not worrying about what General Depression or Colonel Anxiety have planned for their next offensive, not waiting for a shoe to drop, just feeling good, living life compassionately, but in control. I do know that to whatever degree I use self-compassion, it will be in conjunction with meditation and contemplation and introduced at a pace where a degree of institutional control can be maintained. I know that I sound like the dickhead warden at Shawshank Penitentiary but image what would happen if you take people locked up for decades and just open the doors and walk away, what do you think would happen? It would be a circus train hitting the Slipknot tour bus that got stuck on the train tracks. Pandemonium would ensue. I have to guard against injecting self-compassion so quickly that could lead to a loss of discipline, but not withholding it to the point where my subconscious would crawl through a sewer main to escape the constant haranguing. That being said my eyes have been opened wide to how important self-compassion can be if wielded wisely and that in and of itself is a big change for me. A year ago, if told that it was possible, I would have agreed with you while shaking my head no, just so you wouldn't feel bad about saying something so profoundly stupid. Now with the progress, with the meditation and mindfulness, I think at some point with consistent effort, that it just may be possible, and that, my friends, is hope.

MONDAY, JULY 13, 2020

Being optimistic about a Monday morning does not come naturally, I think I talked with you about that, and if I'm being brutally honest, there isn't one day of the week that really jumps out as my favorite anymore, days just stopped trying, and it's sad. I think I have also expressed my opinion regarding happy morning proverb reciters who constantly say things like "look on the bright side" or "it could always be worse" and how I would like to roundhouse kick them right in the earhole. Of course, I would promptly rip my pants, and in the end, they would be correct anyway; there are far worse things than a Monday, starting with flesh eating bacteria, so I rise and hope the "shine" will happen naturally at some point over the course of the day.

I have an immediate opportunity to improve my outlook and start the day productively, but it requires taking the woolly my-mutts on a walk, and since they have gone forty-eight hours without one, they are being super-duper a-holes. There were no deaths or serious injuries on the walk, and we all made it back, so I'm going to declare an early victory and celebrate by drinking some freshly brewed ambrosia water, and revel in small wins. For a long time now, I can't quite remember when I started. I have been breaking the day into bite-size chunks. If I look at the entirety of all that needs to be accomplished, it can be overwhelming, especially when factoring the impact of my depression and the additional mental energy that is takes to keep it in check while moving from activity to activity. Dealing with humans in any capacity during a day can also add an additional degree of unpredictability, since humans are inherently arbitrary in nature requiring my constant attention to be "on guard," and a higher energy output to keep my depression symptoms at bay. The most challenging aspect of any day, the thing that seems to drain energy faster than anything else is the impossible task.

I know when you hear about an "impossible task" and you don't have a depressive frame of reference, your mind may picture a high mountain peak enveloped by clouds, or a race with a far distant finish line, maybe even doing something really cool and not posting about it on social media. You see, the "impossible task" is a depression thing, it has less to do with human achievement possibilities and more to do with the restricting limitations and debilitating hardships that depression holds over its sufferers. It is something that most people could do easily and without a second thought, like filing taxes, cleaning out the garage, or taking the car in for a long overdue oil change. What makes it impossible is the fact that some inexplicable thing, some unknown force is preventing us from the ability to perform this one stupid fucking thing, and it goes beyond frustration; it makes us question the feasibility of ever feeling like a proper functioning adult.

Like many, I assume, my impossible task has changed over time to reflect my status and to-do list. When I was in junior high school and had to write a big end-of-year report, complete with title page, table of contents, footnotes, and some other shit, I couldn't bring myself to write a word. We were given like a month to complete the assignment and it was to represent a big portion of the overall grade, so there was some impetus behind doing a good job. With each day that passed the pressure to start grew greater and greater and though I sat at my desk pen in hand, a blank sheet of paper held in place by me left hand, I couldn't bring myself to begin. There was a new episode of *The Million Dollar Man* that would draw my attention, or maybe I just needed a nap, but there always seemed to be something that was just a tiny bit more important. I did finish the report in the eleventh hour, thanks to intervention from within, or in other words my mother's foot up my ass. So in case you were wondering, the "impossible" comes from our preconception not from reality; it seems impossible, so it is.

For purpose of another example, I once kept my broken-down truck in front of my mother's house for like six months. It wasn't running right, and it had a tire that always went flat, and I couldn't bring myself to get it fixed, so I borrowed my mom's spare car and left the truck where it sat. Now I could use money as an excuse, how I didn't have the funds to put into the repair, and while there was some truth in there it was like using Colonel Steve Austin as an excuse for not writing a report, there was a high bullshit quotient. Again, I overcame the impossible to get the job done, but it took an amazing toll on me psychologically. The mental energy required is extraordinary, again, not to complete the task, but to get out of the starting blocks. The closest thing I can compare it to is climbing a steep sand dune and how every step is labored and burdened and the faster you move, the farther the summit seems to be. Anger gives way to frustration, which gives way to disappointment and hopelessness, and your depression is there, embedded, fighting you every step of the way, fueling your feelings of inadequacy, creating an environment of helplessness.

So what is it, you ask, about the nature and characteristic of those activities that lend themselves to be so difficult to accomplish? That's a great question. Having had many and varied experiences with this phenomenon, I can tell you this much—there is usually a worry or stressor behind the activity. Someone may have not paid taxes in seven years because it's their impossible task, but it started in the first year with worry that they owed more than they were able to pay, and it mushroomed from there. Someone else may have not cleaned out their garage or storage unit in a decade because there are items that once belonged to a long-dead loved one, and they don't want the scab ripped off their fragile emotions. For me, in middle school, my thoughts revolved around darkness, and I thought that would be apparent to everyone through my writing, and my truck symbolized my crumbling beat-up self-image. Keep in mind that depression is an opportunistic vulture that senses our fears and weaknesses and will use any means at its disposal to make us feel that the sweet release of death is preferable to moving forward.

The impossible task is the perfect embodiment of the impact depression can have on a seemingly normal human adult. The task is physically and mentally achievable, but by building on guilt and shame felt by not accomplishing the task in a timely fashion, depression takes the significance and amplifies it beyond our ability to overcome. For people looking from the outside, it may seem like a lack of motivation on our part or, dare I say, even a degree of laziness. There is nothing farther from the truth, but there is no clear explanation that would fully describe the overwhelming challenge that it represents in our life because of the emotional baggage that is tied to it. The closest I can get to explaining to a nonsufferer is to tell them to put on a suit of armor and swim a two-hundred-meter individual medley, knowing that if you fail, your family will watch as your loving pet is fed to the jumping sharks from *Shark Week* and that you might drown.

Like depression, there is no "cure" or "fix" for the impossible task, only treatment. You just can't stop feeling the way you do. All you can do is bring awareness and proactivity to the situation. It is categorically imperative that an awareness of the possibility we are creating one of these tasks exists each time we choose to not do something on the basis of our feelings. Being aware is the first step, the second is always the hardest, and that is doing that "thing" as soon as possible, removing the power that depression holds over you by whatever means necessary, including the asking for help. Now I'm fully aware that asking for help is generally reserved for when we are literally on fire and we can't turn the water spigot due to burned hand flesh, or when we get bitten in the face by a rattlesnake and can't suck the venom out and need someone to, you know, suck our faces. Asking for help or talking in general when we are in the trenches fighting hand to hand with our depression can be an impossible task in and of itself, but I have found it an essential in overcoming this hurdle. Every time I have moved beyond one of these barriers, it was with the help or prodding of someone else. Of course, they didn't realize the situation, and I never told them the struggles I was having. I imagine that if I had opened up and told them, they would have readily agreed to help in any way that they could.

I can't say it enough; open up, talk about what you're going through and what your struggles are, and keep doing it. We have the power to change the stigma associated with depression if we all start a conversation with those closest to us. Let me make this clear, people who suffer with depression can do amazing things. We can think, create, achieve, and be heroes instead of villains. We save lives, help people, and love unconditionally. We simply are made a little differently, so we face different challenges, but that difference should not be kept in a dark closet, should not be something we are ashamed of, it does not make us less. I have found as I walk with my anxiety and depression, year after year, that half of my battle is focused on management and vulnerability, in essence, depression-proofing your life. When you have your first child, what do you do around your house, especially when they age toward mobility? You crawl around the house on hands and knees, looking at the environment from their potential point of view, looking for risks, sharp corners, outlets, and running chainsaws. Collecting cacti was probably a bad choice. You do the same for your depression; look at it from your depressions point of view—what are your weaknesses and what risks do they present?—and assess regularly as your depression will morph and change over time.

I have taught myself to talk about my anxieties and my darkness. I didn't want to at first for being "outed" as different, didn't want to bring anyone into or expose them to what I experience on a regular basis. The plain fact of the matter is that by opening up and being honest, you are helping everyone build a greater understanding of what it means to suffer with depression, and at the same time, you are reducing the weapons it can bring to bear against you. The easiest way to defeat the impossible task is to catch it when it's still just an "I really don't want to do that. I can, but I don't want to" task. It always starts as something you just don't want to do either for emotional or psychological reasons. By depression-proofing your life, you become more aware of when those issues are developing and can defuse them before they become dangerous or simply impossible.

TUESDAY, JULY 14, 2020

Life in the days of COVID-19, a Hollywood triple feature playing concurrently, *Groundhog Day, Contagion,* and *Rocky Horror Picture Show.* You'll cry, you'll cry harder, you'll develop an aversion to pants, then throw up a little in your mouth and need an Altoid. Do you know who loves it? Izzy, Hondo, and Maudie, los tres factorias de mierda; they freaking love that we are all home most of the time, making it convenient for belly rubs and snacks and to witness them doing the thing they love to do most, protecting the house and family by barking at everything that casts a shadow. When normalcy returns and we are able to "go" to work, there will be a collective howl, and all tails will be at half-wag, but for now we're all home doing the best we can do to hold it together. As I leash them up, I hope that cheeky cat that likes to taunt the dogs by acting unimpressed isn't out this morning.

Today is a coffee day. "Coffee all day, party till nine-ish, baby!" I don't do this all the time, but I'm drinking coffee right now, then later this morning, I'm meeting a friend named Joe for another *cup* of joe. I grew up with pots of coffee, like it was a member of our family, which we drank to death. When I worked with my father, he was forever making coffee, and everything was a good reason to brew a fresh pot. "Oh boy, the suns coming out, let's make some coffee" or "I just got this new tie, and nothing goes together with fresh neckwear like fresh coffee." Caffeine runs through my veins and is part of my DNA just as much as blood and the rest of that sciencey shit.

Joe is a great guy. He deals with a degree of depression from time to time, so he has a real basis of understanding when I speak

154

of mine, plus, like me, he's got some miles behind him, so he's been around and done stuff. It is all kinds of therapeutic to talk with another human about life, not just about the depression part, but about sports, or robots taking over the government, which I think we both agreed would be a step in the right direction. We sip good coffee and talk easy as falling down a hill; the minutes fly by. The subject of depression is never broached and that's the best of things. It's fully obvious that neither of us needs to, so we don't. I'm the biggest proponent of talking in the world, literally. I'm just waiting for the call from the Guinness people to confirm and send me a letter or something. That being said, it's not just opening up about depression or feelings. There is a lot of other stuff in the world that needs a good talking about too. Conversation isn't as much about your voice as it is finding your voice.

It is amazing how a person can go weeks and months, have a family, hold down a job, maybe ever volunteer at the food bank, or sing in the church choir and not really "say" anything. I know that I've gone extended periods saying little more than the superficial requirements of polite societal norms. I would say hello, tell people I was "fine," and go about my day saying as few words as possible. I'm sure that people thought I was "off," but nobody pressed or dug deeper because we have created a stigma around asking personal questions that make caring seem rude or invasive. How many times in news reports have we heard that the individual who killed themselves or others labeled as "a quiet person" or that they "preferred to be alone." It was always a fear of mine in the old days, after they found my body, that someone would remember me as a "loner," because I wasn't. I just didn't know how to talk or how to open up to someone else.

Always remember that only whores and politicians jump right into their feelings. You have to warm up to that serious shit. You don't see athletes get right off the bus and immediately start playing or Mike Tyson just wake up and start eating human ears. There's a process in place that will facilitate the preparation, the warming up, the stretching out. You have to approach talking the same way. You start light. The weather is always a good beginner because it's a shared experience. Unless you're starting a conversation on the

International Space Station, you've probably had a run in with the weather today. Then you talk about new shows on whichever streaming service or how your team would have won the trophy for whatever this year if sports were still a thing, before saying "I need to talk about something."

My hour with Joe is coming to an end. We've exhausted our coffee supply and the time allotted, so we say our goodbyes and we make plans to do it again soon. I have a full day ahead of me with work and gym, a lot of reps and calls, sweat and emails. No matter what life and work bring, your responsibilities to yourself go on, and for as long as there is breath in your body, so shall you! I don't know why, but I pictured myself in a suit of armor, standing on a wagon giving a rah-rah speech to a bunch of dirty peasants. There is nothing wrong with the peasants, they're just dirty because nobody had floors back then.

Once I checked all the boxes and called it a day, I decided to turn on the nightly news and get a glimpse of what's going on in the world. I sat down in the fluffy chair with the remains of my last cup of coffee for the day and take a deep cleansing breath while the commercial trying to sell me cream cheese or sour cream or cottage cheese finishes up. Why does dairy make some people so happy? The news comes on and less than five minutes later I'm like running down the hall with my fingers in my ears saying "La, la, la, I can't hear you." Holy shit, reality will fuck your mood right up. When I was a kid my parents were watching a movie late one night. I came downstairs to use the bathroom or get a drink, and the situation piqued my interest. Seeing me, my mom tried shooing me back upstairs, saying, "This is a grown-up movie," obviously unconcerned what future me would think about that statement. I insisted and my father, just wanting the annoying interruption to come to an end, allowed me to stay until the next commercial. I sat between them, under my mom's famous "fear blankie," guaranteed to protect against monsters big and small, and was introduced to a movie called *The Exorcist*. Fifteen minutes later found me walking back up the stairs, visions of creepy girls riding flying beds and head-spinning puke fountains dominated my senses. The rest of that night was spent under my blankets, hearing demonically possessed, highly flexible people walk up the stairs to projectile vomit on me.

The point is that I should have listened to my mom. I should have gotten my drink or peed, then promptly returned to my cozy ignorance. Once you see something, you can't unsee it. There will be no "blue pill" that will allow you to return to your normal life or make your dick hard. I felt that way about the news, just one sad, depressing story after the next, people being assholes, people dying, people being assholes while dying. It literally took the wind out of my sails, figuratively. My mood dropped, my blood pressure began to rise, a change was coming, and I wasn't the only one who noticed, so let's talk about it.

Meditation and contemplation have become a part of my daily routine, so much so that I may gloss over it like some of the other acts of daily living, but rest assured, that it is happening, and it is helping me dramatically, as you are doing by patiently listening. I have been creating a greater overall awareness through mindfulness that is really starting to pay off. Being confronted with negative input, such as "bad news," I see now how it affects me and how I react to it. I see the cues clearly that lead to a downward modulation in attitude, and most importantly, I have begun to see the actions and thoughts forming that are like drops of blood in the water to my ominously circling depression.

This is an amazing tool that I never believed that I would possess, like one of those circular saws with a laser beam that show you where your cutting, because I always start the cut straight, but then it's forever going wonky about halfway through. I can see the damage done, the wound, and take action to heal them before they cost me so much more. Now your mindfulness "Schwartz" may be bigger than mine, and you may feel that you learned in minutes what it has taken me weeks to reach awareness of, and to that I would say "good for you!" but I would say it sarcastically while coughing. I'm getting to the age where I can't remember if I've already talked about something or if I just thought about talking about something, so I appreciate you bearing with me if I've covered this ground before. I know my father would tell the same stories to largely the same audience almost every time he saw them. Nobody ever called him out or said anything, mostly because he was a captivating storyteller, but also out of respect, but I noticed and watched and studied, so it's possible that my apple is sitting right next to his tree trunk and that's just fine with me.

Whether or not I've already covered some of this ground, I think it's vitally important, so I'm going to say some other stuff and hope you will forgive me my redundancy. I'm still a neophyte deep thinker, so when I meditate, I rely on a rote process that I repeat daily. I find a peaceful place with a comfortable seat. Depending on the time of day, the weather, and the disposition of the yapping hyenas, this may be outside or in a closed room. I sit easy and take the stereotypical pose, hands folded into my lap, shoulders relaxed, eyes closed. I don't start immediately. I allow my minds momentum to slow before starting in on my slow, focused breathing. The breaths aren't to work on breathing, which is done automatically. They are to help focus the mind, to employ it in helping reach a deeper level of softened awareness. I know that you probably heard Enya playing during that last part, but the whole idea is to reach a level of concentration where you aren't concentrating on concentration. I've found that it's really hard to explain what you experience, but it's like obtaining focus by losing focus. Shit, why don't you just Google it.

When I do reach that place, I am either going to follow a guided meditation or run my own program. If I'm on my own, I focus on three areas, thoughts, feelings, and actions. Actions are the easiest because unless I punched a nun in the face for not wearing a mask in public. Chances are, I haven't done a lot physically to raise a flashing light to my depression, but I don't cut the corner because one day I might, not punch a nun but something else. Thoughts come next, but first there has to be a distinction between thoughts and feelings because they are closely related. Thoughts are our personal theories or opinions based on known information; feelings are products of our thoughts and experiences. Now I'm not going to lie to you and tell you I can easily categorize my thoughts and feelings as they often bleed together, but it really doesn't matter, as long as I'm giving myself the opportunity to process the negative offenders.

Now I read something somewhere that the average person has fifty to seventy thousand thoughts per day, which seems like way too many, even at the low end of the scale that would be almost thirty-five a minute. Now I'm guessing that many of those are happening unconsciously, behind the curtain, of our operational mind and require no active participation. What I am hoping for is the opportunity to pick a weed in my mental garden before it grows into, I guess, a bigger weed. I don't know a lot about weeds or gardening. I can work through my thoughts and feelings about what I witnessed on the news and what caused me to feel negatively about myself and my environment that increased my overall pessimism about life. In the past, those thoughts and feelings would go untended and grow, providing constant sustenance to my burgeoning depression. By sensing a change in mood and demeanor, then having the ability and taking the time to examine the root causes and determine what changes, if any, I could make to adjust my thought paradigm. I am becoming a better gardener, at least mentally.

I hate gardening, by the way, always have. My version of hell, my regular version, not my depressed version, is that I get there and Beelzebub shows me this vast garden of his favorite vegetables: broccoli, brussels sprouts, and onions, with a spattering of cauliflower. This garden of hell-i-tables seems to go on for miles, and in between the neatly organized massive rows are freckles of weeds dotting the bare ground. Then old man Lucifer looks at me, smiles, and hands me the only tool I will have to assist me, a cracked plastic spork; that's it, not even one of those gel knee pads or frumpy large-brimmed hat to protect my neck from the heat. I would get on my knees and start working around the circumference of the weed with the measly tool provided, gently pulling in order to get roots and all, but at the moment, I try to pull it free of the soil, it would break apart, leaving the roots firmly planted, guaranteeing another would soon grow. Lucifer would laugh at my misfortune while picking vile vegetables and shout, "Wait till you see what's for dinner." When I was a kid, I thought I was being punished for something I had done when I was asked to help weed. I just kept apologizing, hoping at some point to be pardoned and set free to do anything else. I do remember pulling up a new patch of strawberry plants, thinking that they were weeds once, and getting in trouble, but not being asked to help weed again, so it was totally worth it.

To continue with the whole "garden" thing, the more vigilant of a gardener that you are, the better your garden looks and grows, I would assume. By meditating about the general negativity that developed from watching the news, I was able to realize that it led to no adverse actions on my part, and that my thoughts were a result of skewed vision of a world on fire, descending into oblivion. My feelings then became far more pessimistic and hopeless based on that thought pattern. The ability to, one, examine the genesis of a harmful thought cycle and, two, actually deal with it effectively, before it can germinate or develop, has been a sea change in my life. I fucking love it. At the end of the day, I realized that I cannot do anything about the news or the state of affairs of the world. I can control my access to it and how I let it affect me, today and tomorrow. So for now, I'm just going to keep the news turned off. Now you may feel like you need that information on the daily; if that's the case, you do you. I don't choose to be ignorant of important issues forever, just until I'm in a stronger state of mind, and at the end of the day, I would rather be uninformed and at ease than educated and at battle.

I highly recommend that every depression sufferer on the planet and even hypertensive and depressive aliens, self-conscious about their freakishly large heads and ghoulishly long, skinny fingers, should have a daily mindfulness habit. It's totally weird and uncomfortable at first, especially if you're a meathead like me and expect pan-flute music to be playing, incense to be burning in Himalayan salt holder carved in the shape of a dragon, and Sting to be having tantric sex in the corner for like five hours. Work through the initial awkwardness and take time every day. It won't take very long to start seeing a change in how you feel. Don't think that it's a one-and-done either; you can meditate multiple times a day, as much as you feel you need to overcome a difficult situation. The more time you spend, the more you learn; the more you learn, the greater control you experience.

This afternoon's mindfulness session took under fifteen minutes. I'm sure for many people they could do it in less, and it was time very well spent. We all spend time in our day doing random stuff. I'm sure that no matter how busy your day is, you could find ten or fifteen minutes that will give you so much more in return.

WEDNESDAY, JULY 15, 2020

Hey, good morning, my friend. I hope Morpheus was kinder to you than he was to me, having yet another restless sleep cycle. I've been working on shutting down my mind in the middle of the night, to varying degrees of success. I find it funny, not men wearing capris pants funny, more Sonic the Hedgehogs given first name is Ogilvie funny, that attempting to meditate during sleeping hours actually stimulates me beyond the ability to rest. I'm going to treat last night as a failed experiment that garnered valuable information in lieu of success. I now know more than I did yesterday and will gladly trade sleep to get a hold of my depression. That being said, a tired me is a vulnerable me, so I can't string too many nights like this together.

I get out of bed and start revolving with the earth, "once more into the fray." The three canine-tastrophies get walked and fed, and I'm able to spend some quality time with a hot mug of velvety rich liquid mahogany that warms the cuckolds that live in my heart. I sit with Lisa and go over what this day holds. I'm a big fan of having a plan, especially if it involves a van filled with flan and a man named Dan. Suck it, Eminem. A plan gives structure to the day. It provides marching orders and encompasses what needs to be done and what we would like to do if time allows.

In the past four months, Lisa and I have spent more time together than in a normal year, and while many family therapists and divorce lawyers are putting down payments on vacation homes in Vail or the Mexican Riviera, we have found that we are highly compatible and can spend extended periods of time together, which is a plus while on quarantine, or if we both have to go to the DMV. Lisa

162

is a school bus driver by trade. I may have mentioned that earlier. I can't remember because of the sleep thing. Being a school bus driver means that on any given weekday, when school is attended, she is up early, getting her fitness in, prepping her snack and lunch, getting cleaned up, and heading out, often before the sun's at full power. I'll be honest in telling you that some mornings after she leaves, I will lie on the couch and nod off while Noah watches Animal Planet shows, at least until the fourth ASPCA commercial in a row comes on and I can't take it anymore. Since the pandemic, Lisa and her compatriots have been dry-docked, which has changed practically everything but the routine.

So we spend most waking hour in each other's presence, which I have absolutely no problem with at all. Lisa, on the other hand, may feel slightly different. I tell her that this is our dry run for retirement, but I think to myself, "If this is what retirement is going to be like, then it's looking boring as fuck." One of the biggest challenges that we face on a daily is just staying motivated to move forward, at least for her, with a job but no work, with many activities still closed or inaccessible. Some days having nothing to do seems like a welcome respite from the grind, but when you string days and weeks of idleness together, it becomes the grind, an obstacle that needs to be hurdled every day.

Let's talk for a little bit about what it's like to go through a dramatic period of history, with historic stresses and mounting daily difficulties while suffering with depression. The easy answer is that it fucking sucks, but let's dive a little deeper, shall we? People with depression, and by people I'm referencing a large number of people, and by depression I'm referencing the full range of depressive disorders and the varying degrees in which they affect the previously referenced large number of people. Let's agree that each person's depression is a unique and individual combination of circumstance and affliction that makes them like no other. We sufferers are all distinctive arches, loops, and whorls experiencing the spectrum of misery, so when I talk about depression sufferers, it covers a vast cross-section of humanity.

I believe wholeheartedly that there are advantages and disadvantages to being depressed on lockdown. I hate assholes who ask, "Do you want the good news or bad news first?" Only lighthouse keepers and panderers want the good news first. Everyone else wants the happy ending, in every sense of the words. That being said, let's look at the disadvantages associated with the interplay between depression and quarantine from my point of view. I would say that the most prodigious disadvantage is that bad news and sheltering in place feel a lot like walking into a stadium where you're the visitor and the seats are packed with people wearing "Go Depression" jerseys, and upon seeing you, a chorus of "boos" rain down. Then, here comes your depression and everyone goes crazy. Even the referees are cheering madly, which you find odd. The sheer amount of negativity and degree of loss of control are hard to overcome if you are unencumbered with a depressive disorder but becomes almost debilitating when coupled with the darkness.

It's no secret that depressed people tend to withdraw when in an active fight, so there is a prevailing school of thought that this may be an actual advantage that sufferers have over the nondepressed population. I disagree, again speaking in generalities. When we withdraw or self-isolate it is a management tool that allows a degree of manipulation over the time we control. We still rely on outside stimulus to hold on to a degree of normalcy, going to work, getting a coffee at a coffee shop, being around other humans and having contact by proxy. While you think quarantine would play right into our hands, like everyone else we still need contact and connection and suffer without it.

Kind of on the same lines is the loss of routine. Like myself, many people who deal with depression rely on a firm, predictable routine to get through the dark days. Functional depressives need to know what's coming next; there has to be a structured game plan and associated timeline. We will develop our routines and rote "muscle memory" activities to a degree that when we are on a down cycle. Otto the Pilot can kick in and get us through with minimum inputs on our behalf. When routines change, and there is no positive association, like if you were to take a vacation to Maui, it can have a significant impact. All of a sudden, having people around that aren't normally or being deprived of places and things that held a substantial importance can lead to new lows and darkening outlooks.

There normally aren't benefits to a depression diagnosis. There's no 401(k), the coffee in the breakroom is both instant and decaf, and the company car is a hearse that you only get to ride in once. The biggest advantage to living with depression during times of crisis is dealing with elements of the bizarre. We see things that others don't in a way that they can't imagine, so in dealing with situations with that dark, surreal quotient, we have a real advantage. If the world suddenly turned monochromatic and a vast army of Sasquatch that had been amassing and training in terrorist warfare in tight cells in heavily wooded areas around the globe started to cut people's heads off demanding free Wi-Fi access, we would shrug and think, "Yeah, that sounds about right." Many of us see darkness and dark things. Many others feel the darkness around them. Regardless, we are uniquely suited to dealing with hard shit.

We live with hard shit we see and feel on the daily, above and beyond the "normal" hard shit life throws at us from time to time. Day in and day out, working, grinding it out, so in addition to our ability to handle it, we can handle it for a long time, which brings me to perhaps the greatest advantage, stamina. We are comfortable spending "time under tension." If the shit-show lasts two years or twenty years, we bought the ticket, and we'll take the ride. Most people look at the lockdown as a major inconvenience that will last a period of time. It sucks and then at some point it will be over. People with depression are in a fight every fucking day, regardless of what the world is throwing at them. We are battle-hardened but not masochistic. If indeed that there was an "easy button" in life, that bitch would be worn out, but we know that there isn't and our fight will be there tomorrow, and the next day, and long after COVID-19, it is just a footnote in the history books, if they still bother making those things.

The deal is, nobody is going to emerge from this period of time unscathed, and nobody is going to receive a trophy for winning. We will all lose someone or something that we hold dear, and some will lose everything. For many, depressed or not, this period of time will prove too much, and they will lose their fight, they will succumb to the negativity, and they will take their lives, and that is a tragedy. This whole train of thought wasn't to show that depressed people will inherit the earth after all the "normies" run off a cliff chasing the Grubhub delivery guy, or to say that in a crisis the nuclear launch codes should be entrusted to the most clinically depressed person alive, I was merely trying to point out that there are times when a negative can indeed be a positive. More than anything, I would love to see people sharing, sharing their strengths and their struggles, people suffering with long-term depression standing up and talking, guiding the new, situationally induced depressives through their differing emotions, locking arms with their community to ensure no one has to die feeling alone. This is how we work together to rid ourselves of the stupid stigma that surrounds mental illness that makes people feel they are resigned to a shadowy existence. Okay, sorry, I got a little fired up there. I really wanted to flip the kitchen table, but you know, Lisa.

I fucking hate when people kill themselves because of feelings. If you're an asshole who's done bad things and can't live with it, that's someone else's department. My mission, my passion is to put an end to the senseless and totally preventable deaths that occur because of little more than difficulty in communication. Communication is the viscous oil that keeps the machine that is our existence, purring along and not grinding to a halt. Before you go there, know that I know that this has been brought up. This is not one of those times that I tell you I can't remember if I've said something, I know for a fact we've gone over this, but I need to say shit twenty-eight times before it sinks in. Why do you think the Bible tells you not to boink the other people in every chapter? If you or someone you know is having a tough time communicating for the love of God, and the sake of my blood pressure, please start talking, and if that seems unreasonable, find another human and start listening. This will 100 percent save lives if we all do it, people will not feel alone or hopeless if they know that there are others who feel similarly, and there is hope, of connection and belonging, but you have to create it.

Jesus, I just get so tired of the insecurity bullshit, that depression is outside societal norms and should be treated as such. I never apologize for going off about opening up and shedding light on dark issues. I would rather be criticized for being too loud than regret being too silent. All right, the blood pressure has returned to normal. I have put my soapbox away for the moment and I'm searching for a way to less awkwardly transition to something else. Since I was young and there was an uncomfortable moment or lull in the conversation, I would always think to myself, "Let's talk about my dick," and it would always make me smile because it would most likely be inappropriate and nongermane, but I would smile, and people would wonder why. It's stupid, I know, but it's me. I'm actually smiling right now.

We found ourselves in the afternoon without afternoon stuff to do, so I asked Lisa for her input, which was a tactical error on my part. I knew when her eyes lit up that it wasn't going to involve actual fun. "I want to go to the dump and get rid of all the cardboard." Goddammit. It shouldn't have surprised me in the slightest. She has hated Boxemite (pronounced like *Yosemite*, only with *Box* instead of *Yos*) since I created it and commemorated it just after Christmas 2019. Boxemite was formed naturally by breaking down cardboard boxes and stacking them under the carport next to the garbage and recycling bins. There was, in actuality, way too much to fit into our bimonthly recycling bin, so the idea was to stack it up, and through the normal recycling process over time, Boxemite would experience geologic erosion until there would be nothing left. Suddenly, El Capi-Rona erupted and overnight everything was coming in boxes and ending up on the pile. Boxemite grew impressively but, in doing so, made it hard to navigate under our car-less carport with our broken clothes dryer, broken gas barbecue, and collection of empty spray-paint cans. The monument to capitalism had to go, and apparently today was the day.

I'm just going to say this: I hate spiders, and there is no reasonable basis for my dislike other than I just can't abide spiders. Before you tell me how beneficial they are to the environment and they keep bug populations in balance and shit, know this, unless they find me a huge tax loophole, or save my child's life that, they are my sworn nemesis. That being said, do you have any idea, besides liquefied bug guts, what spiders love? You're right, cardboard freaking boxes. I felt like Indiana Jones a little today, but instead of snakes and Nazis, it was spiders, and instead of the ark of the covenant, I discovered was that I could fit all the majesty of Boxemite in the back of the truck, and that having a spider crawl on me makes me pee a little.

I start up the truck, and Lisa and Noah load up, to help out and to get out of the house for a little while. As we make the twenty-min-ute drive to the junk-processing center, my mind recalls when I used to love going to the dump. When I was a kid, the dump was just this big field that you would go and literally just dump your crap on the ground or in the piles that would be formed by the dozers con-stant attention. I used to love going there and just wandering around, finding little treasures that the original owner didn't, um, treasure. I could spend hours picking through other people's crap, and just as soon as I wrote that, I realized it doesn't sound as romantic a notion as it actually was. Back in the day when kids actually built stuff and used authentic imagination in their play, that place was a goldmine just waiting, um, to be mined. Alas, my mother forbade me bringing home more than we were dumping, because, well, it was garbage, but a few items made it through inspection, hidden in the deep pockets of my Lee Rider corduroy pants or in my "keister." Just kidding, I didn't learn how to "keister" until I went to church camp in high school and couldn't live without my Walkman.

Eventually the "open pit" method of trash depositing gave way to the more convenient and hygienic method of dumping your crap at a transfer station that was located closer to town. Now you just back the truck up to a wire fence overlooking a massive concrete pit. Both sides were lined with vehicles of all shapes and sizes raining unwanted discards to the pit floor below, where an enormous bull-dozer would compact it and move it ever forward to be processed further and sent to the dump proper. My current greatest "dump" activity is to take the heaviest thing I'm dumping and throw it at the most breakable thing I can find on the pit floor. I've found out some cool stuff in the process, like the old cathode tubes in bygone television sets are really hard to break, and that if you hit them just right, spray paint cans will kinda explode, which is awesome. I once broke a toilet by hitting it with another toilet, and that was super satisfying. Today's visit was going to be far less fun because all I had was cardboard and some wood castoffs, and they don't go into the "pit," they go in their own dumpsters that offer no visceral feedback when stuff is thrown into them.

At the end of the day, it cost me a total of seven dollars and forty-five cents, some time, and a case of the heebie-jeebies, but getting out of the house and putting a semi-smile on Lisa's face was worth every penny. I'm going to head home and meditate and spend some time working on the upstairs, meaning my brain. I'm going to try and figure out a way that I can once again let people know how I feel about talking through depression and being an active participant. I just don't know how to facilitate it or promote it to the masses. I absolutely believe with my entire heart and soul that suicide caused by depression can be eliminated, that all people can experience hope, can feel the sun on their faces and smile. We have the power within us to make this happen. If you feel broken and useless, please know this—you are not garbage; you are vital and important and will one day realize that, if you stick around.

THURSDAY, JULY 17, 2020

I haven't wanted to bring it up because while I'm not superstitious, I hold this belief that's not based on reason or knowledge but on the ominous significance of a particular thing, but knock on wood, I haven't had a bout of PTSD in almost two weeks. This came to mind when I was having a meditation session this morning and was really focusing on positive thoughts, not specific to the PTSD but just general, natural positivity. Now I'm not a medical professional of any kind, but I really could have been but apparently lacked the requisite interest in mathematics and science shit. Regardless of my medical inexperience, I still feel two weeks symptom free is a success, not a cure, but definitely movement in the right direction. I know, I'm not superstitious but I just threw salt over my left shoulder, put away my Ouija board, and responded to a chain letter just because it was the right thing to do.

I'll tell you my reasoning behind how I have been attacking my PTSD, which isn't really an attack at all, because PTSD doesn't exist. Calm down, let me explain. PTSD is as real as that super-long hair on my nipple, but it's not real all the time. My mind conjures it up based on past experiences and current environmental inputs. It is, for lack of a better term, a ghost in the machine. All of the elements that make up my PTSD are in my mind somewhere as thoughts, just waiting to be set free by an external trigger that, in my case, can't be avoided. So I approach it the same way I approach my depression exposure management. I am not trying to cure myself forever, because at this point of non-*Star Trek* medicine, it's not possible, but to get to a point that I could live with it forever and do so success-

170

fully. Honestly, my daily routine is not designed around or specifically mandated for the treatment of PTSD. At this point I don't even know what a genuine "treatment" would look like, but by actively managing my anxiety and depression, there seems to be a carryover element to the PTSD. That leads me to conclude what I originally suspected, that the triumvirate of anxiety, depression, and PTSD is closely related, with overlapping spheres of effect and treatment. I have absolutely no clue if this is correct. I just wanted to sound smart, and frankly, it didn't make me feel as good as I had hoped.

When I experience an episode of PTSD, it is all about anxiety; it exudes it through my pores. But it's not like my generalized anxiety about seemingly everything else; it's like my anxiety took a blast of gamma radiation to the face, and when it gets mad, it turns into some Incredible Hulking anxiety that just wants to smash shit before returning to my normal anxiety and roaming around waiting for something to piss it off again. That is why I feel so strongly about my efforts to rid myself of anxiety, why the mindfulness stuff is so important right now, because it deals with the root causes of my anxiety. For so long I have focused almost exclusively on the depression, trying to keep it from killing me, letting the anxiety run naked through my mental fields and rub its junk all over my nice plants or whatever. In allowing it to operate outside the law I feel I have created a welcoming environment for PTSD, so in keeping with that line of reasoning, if I start clubbing my anxiety over the head with a two by four and running it out of town, it should have a positive effect on the PTSD. What time will tell is what impact the absence of overwhelming anxiety will have on my depression. My hope is that the less anxiety I have to deal with, the greater awareness I can bring to bear in my fight with depression, which should even out the playing field somewhat.

I'm feeling pretty good about the progress I've made and the work I've put in, so I give myself a rare pat on the back. Of course, not literally because I have the shoulder mobility of brick fireplace. It feels good to allow the "positive vibes" about myself without thinking I'm going soft or losing my edge. To keep the party atmosphere that only I can feel, a rockin' I decide that it is a perfect summer day to pull out the stand-up paddleboard and kayak that have been keeping the dust off our shed floor and see if they still float after being dry-docked all of last summer. I drag them around the house and throw them in the back of the truck. It is a Deevers family tradition, handed down through generations, directing that whatever the load. It should be so tightly secured that it takes an inordinately long period of time to untie once you reach your destination. My dad was in the Navy, and back then in between killing whales, or whatever the fuck the Navy does, I guess they would sit around and tie sheepshanks and bowlines. He knew all the knots and would tie stuff down to such a degree that it was a feasible possibility you'd forget what you were doing in the first place by the time he was done untying the knots. I don't know knots, but I do like tying stuff down, in the bed, of the truck. I have thought about it and there is no way to desexualize that last sentence.

I know that when the knot looks like it was tied with kitchen beaters that the boats were acceptably secured. I'm not as much driven by the satisfaction of doing the job properly as by the nightmare vision of the boats falling out and pinballing around the interstate hitting one litigious driver after the next. I grab the life jackets, Lisa, and Noah, and we hit the road. We're heading for the same lake that we rode our bikes around last week, so we have a thirty-minute drive. We find the park inhabited but not overly so, definitely fewer people than the weekend, which was a plus. Here's a life hack for all of you who like to tie something so poorly that it looked like you did it with kitchen beaters: keep some scissors handy and just cut the rope. Seriously, life's too short and rope is not that expensive. Cut the shit and move on with your day. In each corner of my truck bed is a metal loop, for the express purpose of having a place to tie off. Each one of those loops has rope fragments of varying length and age, representing stuff I've secured since 2007, it's like a woven time capsule of shame, as my father would have disapproved, citing "it's not a proper knot unless it can be untied."

Once freed of their captivity, we walk the boats down the boat ramp to the lapping water's edge and gently sit them down. I run back to the truck to grab the paddles and the life vests, excitement welling up within me. It has been some time since I've been afloat, and I am really looking forward to it. Noah will go on the water but not all the time. Today he prefers to watch from shore, so we get him set up with a chair and some water in a nice shaded spot overlooking the lake. Being the gentleman I am, I give Lisa the first option, sit or stand, and she chooses the standup paddleboard, which makes me happy because I suck on that thing.

It's all about balance. If you lead a good life and are pure of heart, you can stand up and paddle even on the windiest of days, and today is warm and breezy. Lisa paddles out to deeper water on her knees, reaches stabilization, and rises, one leg at a time. I can't help but draw a comparison between her standing on the water and the last month of my life. There I am, just living life, thinking I've got a firm grasp of reality, then a series of events unfold that shake me to my foundation and I fall, hard. Even though there is always a choice to stay down or get back up, I have never given myself a vote. I will get up or meet my end in the attempt. I worked hard, rebuilt my foundation, sought help, learned, grew, and regained my stability. I took care of myself both physically and mentally. My hands come off the board and grasp the paddle. From here I can function, can adjust heading even begin to enjoy life to a degree again. As I continue to gain strength, I become acclimated to the way the water moves and can slowly raise myself to a standing position. Because I've done it correctly, taken time, and made an honest effort, I can stand with a degree of comfort, but I must remember that with every success is sown the seeds of imminent failure, so I must remain constantly vigilant and make adjustments and shift balance to avoid the next fall.

I like this metaphor for a couple of reasons. The first is that it makes me seem like a deep thinker, which makes people not want to fight me, and two, there are tie-ins or other psychological angles you could relate to the core principles, such as wake. "Don't let the wake of someone else's boat make you fall off yours." That needs work but is accurate. You could tie in getting professional help by upgrading the equipment, which also needs work, but I think this metaphor has legs. Now I get the irony, great metaphor about me getting back on my feet after falling, but it's not me on the board, it's Lisa, and she hasn't fallen. I know I'm taking liberties here, but it doesn't goddamn work if the extent of my paddle-boarding ability is looking like a performer in Disney's *Crackheads on Ice: The Musical.*

I rein in my mind and become present in the moment. I'm sitting in a kayak on a lake on a warm summer afternoon, paddling along, listening to the waves gently slap the outside of my craft as I work along the shoreline. I may not be able to conjure up a fancy metaphor with a kayak in it, but if you could sit in my seat right now, the warmth of your skin kissed by a cool eastern breeze, the sparkle of a thousand tiny waves in the distance, and a horizon filled with lush green trees and white-tipped mountains beyond, you would feel, if only for the briefest of moments, what peace feels like. In this instant I have alleviated my anxiety, my depression has been cured, and I am master of the universe!

Unfortunately, I can't live on a kayak, and magic moments often don't last longer than it takes you to say abracadabra, but I have a smile on my face, and I feel alive and functioning, so I don't need to classify it, don't need to stick it in a scrapbook or make a Facebook post, it's my moment and I'm better for having it. We pull into the boat ramp, take off the life vests, and just smile like idiots. It has been a successful adventure, and I'm thirsty and ready to head home. We drag the boats up the ramp and to the truck where Noah is waiting, and I get them tied up with the same precision and attention to detail as on our trip here.

Soapbox time, people. I'm pulling it out and fixin' to orate a spell so if you've been holding it and need to pee or want to pop a Hot Pocket in the Nuker, now would be an appropriate time. Do not underestimate the power of just being outdoors or the therapeutic value that it offers. Go take a walk, or a hike, which is like a walk but longer and your shoes get dirtier, go climb a tree, or ride a bike. The activities are only limited to your imagination, and if there are mosquitos, because if those flying devil fleas are around count me out. Let's perform an experimental study that will never be published. I would like you to perform three activities, each for exactly thirty minutes, and as soon as you complete them, I would like for you to assign a number somewhere on the scale of one, "time to call a hotline," to ten, "I believe I can fly," based on your mood directly after. The three activities are watching the news, trolling Facebook, and taking a walk. I shouldn't have used the term "trolling" for Facebook; it sounds prejudicial, but I don't know what to call it. Watching?

Regardless, be honest and do all three activities at some point over the next few days and see what your numbers are. If your mood isn't significantly better after taking the walk, then maybe you didn't do it right or maybe my methodology is flawed, but hey, you got a walk in, and that's something. In all honesty I set you up, I skewed the activities to prove my point, there is no scientific way that watching news or Facebook could make you feel better than being outdoors. There are multiple studies that have been done linking watching news to deepening depression, and there's even a thing called the Facebook paradox linking users to more stress and anxiety. Apparently by seeing every other human being on earth doing more, seeing more, zip-lining, and bitching about masks is not good for your psyche. If you're a nerd and need a source, type it in your Google box. I don't do footnotes because of formatting. Depression loves media in general. Whether it's news or social, it's not there for your edification; it's there for entertainment. If you learn anything from me, besides you need to talk more, and drink more goddamn coffee, I want it to be that your depression wants to kill you, using your own hands to do it, and will leverage anything you hold dearly important to make that happen.

If you develop insecurities about your life compared to others, your depression will use that against you, and for what? A popularity contest? People whoring out their precious memories and deepest thoughts to fake friends for payment in attention. Have I done it? Hell yes, I have posted pictures with the sole purpose of inciting jealousy and have manufactured an image that isn't always accurate to how I think or feel, and I have paid dearly for creating an inflated importance of it in my own life. There are psychological buttons deep in our reptilian mind that get pushed by social media, and we are seemingly powerless against it, like lab rats masturbating whenever the researchers play an N-Sync song.

Whoa, sorry, I got a little fired up and went "off-script." What the hell was I even talking about? Oh, right, getting outside. Deep breath, focus on the inhale, bringing the mind back, bringing the mind back, focus on the exhale. It is a proven fact that being outdoors reduces stress, lowers anxiety, and leads to feelings of well-being, and not just proven by me when I go outdoors, proven by people with long white coats with their names embroidered on the left side, just above the pocket—embroidered! Now, I'm severely impacted by depression. I'm EFD (every fucking day), so I know that every silver lining is hiding a really cool dark cloud, and that even positive things can be used against us in our minds. "If being outside makes you happier, why don't homeless people smile more?" Or "why would I want to go outside and feel better just to come in and feel worse?" These is the part that nondepressives simply don't understand. They feel that if something makes you feel better, you do that thing and you feel better, get your haircut, put on some nongrayscale clothing, and rejoin the ranks of functioning society.

The truth of the matter is, when we are suffering, hope and relief are very dangerous and very often lead to suicide. Let me explain. I have been to levels in my mind, so dark, so evil that I plainly could not bear the thought of feeling relief for even a moment, fearing the letdown or absence of that relief would be more than I could tolerate. If this is where you are, I would encourage you to seek a greater degree of professional help as soon as possible and Godspeed. For those who are suffering at a more controllable level, I highly recommend the development of a daily outdoor habit of some sort, come rain or shine. Taking a walk, if you're able, is one of the easiest ways to start, get outside, and just move around. I'm being kinda weird about this because, again, short of dirt diving one fathom down, I have been at every possible level of depression, and I know how hard it can be to go down a new road or start a new routine. The depression resists change and will get all up in your head about starting anything. It will discount its value or generate a series of excuses that will sound legit.

I just want to say that at the end of the day it is your life, and it's the only one you're going to get. There won't be a time where someone gives you a "life audit" and goes through your file and says, "Well, it looks like we've severely overfunded your depression account and that you shouldn't have had to deal with that much, so we are going to stop those deposits immediately and give you unlimited carb intake and a baby otter named Chuck." This is your fight, you may have a thousand people in your corner, but when the bell dings, you will be alone in the ring going back into battle. The best fighters work hard on both body and mind, take every opportunity, use every tool, and study and know their opponent. Getting outside, outside your head and the environment you constantly find yourself in is important. Not just important for the standard reasons of reducing stress and anxiety, but important because it gives you some respite, a break from the drudgery that we often find ourselves in, and it's super easy to do.

I'm going to end this for today. I feel I've tilted to the manic as the day has progressed, and I apologize for losing focus and weaving through my thoughts and words like a drunken, hallucinating bumper-car driver. I get enthusiastically overwrought in my thinking and want to vomit everything on the paper to see if anything coherent actually remains. I have given a lot of thought to deleting the whole day and just telling you that my brain was wiped clean by the government or that I bought some ceviche from this guy with no shirt outside fish processing plant and was in the bathroom all day. Upon further thought, I realized that this is who I am. Somedays I can function and communicate clearly; other days I don't feel like I can connect two dots without a protractor. So I will show the good, the bad, and the ugly and hope that you gleaned a kernel of something useful from a pile of shit.

Friday, July 17, 2020

I know that my time with you is coming soon to an end. I can't go on like this forever. I have work to do; you have a life outside listening to me go on and on. Honestly, I didn't think that I would ever make it this far, having spent more time talking with you than all my previous attempts in expressing my feelings combined. I think that my plan right now is to go through my upcoming session with Dr. K, which will probably be the last biweekly meeting with her, barring any setbacks, knock on my wooden head. I will look to connect with her after that on a monthly or bimonthly basis as a way to maintain the progress I have experienced. This is something that I would never, ever have done in the past, but I have seen the value of this process, especially in the "readiness" to participate in a process of stabilizing and advancing personal mental health.

So while this may be the twilight of our time together, Bella. I obviously have a few more things I would like to talk over with you before our paths diverge, and I would like to start by stating for the record that the *Twilight* movies that I referenced overnight wiped out all of the progress and legitimization that the vampire genre had made since *Nosferatu*. There is something about vampires that appeals to people suffering with depression. Maybe it's the aversion to natural light at times, or that we prefer to wear shades of black while avoiding holy water and mirrors, because when we're struggling, we don't care about our hair. Regardless, I need to lock it down and get ready because I'm giving a business Zoom presentation to the Chamber of Commerce about my business and why you should work with me, and I can't be fixated on why vampires just don't use their power and influence to open a blood bank. I mean how easy would it be to form a 501c3 organization, get some volunteers to collect blood during the day, you show up after dark, drink your fill, and send what's left to the hospital, Holy shit look at the time!

I don't just tell people about the pudding, I eat the pudding too, meaning I don't tell people to open up about their mental health experiences from behind the curtain, I have been talking about my struggles within the local business community for years. I don't lead with that as my tagline, and it's not on my business cards, but if there is an opportunity to bring awareness, I will take it. Given that today I am presenting to a bunch of business people and doing so through a PowerPoint via Zoom screen share there is a strict protocol in place for presenters such as me. Everything someone would find offensive should be removed from the home screen, which is fucking impossible nowadays, and the presentation should be no more than twenty minutes and begin with a bio. I start by deleting all booby files from my desktop, and then have a rabbi a priest and a voodoo doctor bless my computer and certify it as fit for human vision. I have several variations of the same bio to accompany the obligatory headshot that I will use from time to time depending on the situation. I hate them all because they are written in the third person and I felt like a conceited d-bag when I was writing them: "Rodger has been in business for over two decades. Rodger likes long walks outdoors because of their therapeutic value. Rodger also likes cheese."

The one thing that the bio gives me is the opening to preach my message: "In his spare time, Rodger likes to bring awareness to depression in the workplace." It gives me a chance to tell people that while I'm sorry that in addition to the stress of running a business, you have to suffer from depression, it's okay that you suffer from depression, and that you are not alone. When your credibility is your business, so many times we hide our depression from everyone, especially the people that we work for and with. We have very real fear that we will lose not only integrity but confidence in our ability and, sooner or later, business. I hid my affliction from anyone and everyone that I could, so when I was having image issues, they were compounded by the energy it took to hide a secret, and as far as secrets go, suffering from depression has got to be the lamest, juiceless secret out there.

Depression will never be a popular workplace topic, because it's fucking depression, I get that, and there is no changing it. What I hope to do, however, is to take on any misconceptions about depression in the workplace and allow people to live feely as who they are and be supported in that effort. "Depressed people will go crazy at some point and do something dramatic." Let's get this straight. Crazy people will do crazy shit, but depression does not equal crazy. There was an unfortunate time, before modern understanding, when depression was "cured" by electroshock, or drilling brain holes, or injecting chemicals into the body or mind, which would forever alter a person's attitude and behavior for the worse. There are endless chilling stories of people with depression who entered asylums and were experimented on until they became clinically insane. Nowadays, though depression may play a part, people do practically the same thing to themselves by injecting worse chemicals into their bloodstream, bringing the asylums to Main Street USA, not the street where you walk into Disneyland and get caramel apples and Mickey-shaped cookies, actual Main Streets, across America.

Depression has always been a convenient scapegoat when talking about erratic behavior, and I'm not going to stand here and tell you that depressed people never act erratically. Shit, I've been institutionalized and once at a crowded "family friendly" event I drunkenly told one of the hosts that if he "didn't get more chicken taquitos I will come back and fuck you in the ass!" Erratic behavior is not under the sole purview of depression. There are many conditions from erectile dysfunction to falling in love that make people do things that they wouldn't normally, which is the very definition of "erratic." The thing is that when a human snaps and does something horrible, the media would rather talk about the bouts of depression, not that he couldn't get his dick hard with cement and rebar, which stigmatizes depression even more. I don't hear the media doing stories about tater tots even though they are clearly responsible for contributing to diabetes and vascular disease, and do you know why? Because they are cute, like little baby potatoes and delicious, with cheese.

I did look this one up for all you "source nerds," according to the National Institute of Mental Health in 2016 over sixteen million people had a major depressive episode, that number represents 7 percent of the population of our country, and those are just the ones that were reported, meaning a form of some kind was filled out. I would say that number is probably light and that it's probably closer to 10 percent of the population. Regardless, the point that I wanted to make was that in 2013, there wasn't sixteen million instances of people going "crazy." Most depression sufferers do so in silence, hiding their issues from the world and, sadly, from support and acceptance. I find it interesting that the actual word "crazy" comes from the English word "craze," which means cracked, or full of cracks, generally used when describing glass, porcelain, or earthenware pottery in the seventeenth century. I don't know why I find that interesting, which in and of itself is interesting.

Let me take a moment to discuss "crazy" in a little more depth. What's the mental image you conjure when you hear that someone went "crazy"? If you're like most people, your mind brings up pictures of horrible mass shootings and loners wanting to inflict as much pain and suffering as possible before cowardly leaving this world. Now I'm not here to argue that those asshats haven't dealt with depression of some degree, but broadly categorizing depressed people because of the extreme actions of a few does a disservice to us all. In a 2016 study by American Psychiatric Association, authored by James Knoll, MD, and George Annas, MD, MPH—wow, two sources in a row—elucidated the fact that mass shootings by people diagnosed with a mental illness represented less than 1 percent of all yearly gun related homicides.

There seems to be another misconception that somehow depressed people may not be as trustworthy as someone who is not depressed. I'm sure that this belief is also tied to the crazy angle, but let's drive down this road anyway. I've been in the financial services industry for the best part of thirty years. I have helped clients make critical decisions that impacted their lives and have held sway over assets large and small, during good times and bad. The thought of taking five cents not owed to me is repulsive. In my darkest of days, in my lowest of lows, I have never been a thief, never dishonored a business commitment or given anyone any reason to lose faith in my ability to do my job in a way constant with the best practices and integrity of my industry.

I am not alone. There are surgeons dealing with depression whose hands right now are in someone else's guts, who will honor the oath they made regardless of their feelings. Overhead there's a pilot who feels the effects of seasonal affective disorder but will ferry his passengers safely and professionally to their destination. There is an engineer who was diagnosed with bipolar depression who designs safety systems for large municipalities. Your life, your health, and your finances have been in depressed hands almost on a daily basis for years. How does that make you feel? What if I were to tell you that the things you hold dear are in the hands of people so strong that they can deal with often terrible personal feelings and still successfully perform their jobs with honor and reliability, feel better? If not, think about this: every day you put your life in the hands of people you don't know. If you are in a car, do think that quarter inch of paint on the road will keep that one-and-a-half-ton car barreling toward you at forty-five miles per hour from hitting you? Remember this, a few years ago, 7 percent of the cars on the road were driven by depressed people.

Now that you know that every day you encounter and trust depressive people in one way or another, wouldn't you want them to work in an environment where they can be supported, accepted, and valued not despite of their affliction but because of it? I would love for people to be able to come forward courageously and be rewarded, not shunned or treated differently. Depression, as it turns out, is as much a medical issue as a psychological issue and shockingly not caused by "bad humors," witches, or back-alley dealings with dwellers of the infernal regions, and it's time we started acting like it. I would like to be a part of ushering in a new era where everyone who suffers can stand and tell their story. If we all do it, we can end the negative stigma that people who suffer with mental illness are cracked and defective.

Again, I am ridiculously transparent with my life and what I've gone through. I don't hold anything back, not for the purpose of garnering attention or sympathy for myself but in hopefully adding to a growing general awareness. You have no idea the number of people who have approached me because of my openness about the struggles they have had or those of loved ones. We are, in essence, doing our depression a favor by keeping it hidden from view. It loves the dark and gains strength from our reluctance to bring the situation to light. Please understand that I am not trying to say in any way that talking about depression cures depression, but living in the light, talking about your feelings, and seeking and finding understanding and support make it so much easier for the sufferer and so much harder on the depression.

While over the years I've given presentations to practically every demographic known to man, and practically most audience sizes from one to five hundred, today will be my first one done virtually, solely reliant on technology. I'm not in the slightest nervous about giving the presentation. I'll do it wearing a speedo while riding a unicycle. I'm fairly nervous about the technological aspects of screen sharing, glitching PowerPoint, low bandwidth kicking me out of Zoom, and Max Headroom "high-tech" goat-fuckery that I've personally witnessed over the last few months.

I sign on to the meeting and there are already twenty people in the "room" networking, which another way to say talking shit, friendly banter, or just catching up. My part of this rodeo doesn't happen for thirty minutes. First, there will be opening remarks then announcements followed by self-introductions, so I settle in. I don't have one of those fancy-pants lifting desktops that allow you to stand and work when your ass deflates, so I use a four-dollar plastic storage box I picked up at Walmart to put under my laptop. It does the job just fine, and the way I see it, you're either going to be all the way up or all the way down. I'm not going to hold a three-quarter squat for thirty minutes. I know it's getting close, and I can talk way better if I'm standing and can use my arms, I don't know why, so I "lift" my computer and give my opening a run through in my head. Opening remarks set the tone and will engage the audience or send them scurrying to the comfort of their phone screens. If you shit the bed and don't set the hook, you might as well be giving a slideshow about a road trip through Nebraska to see the world's biggest goiter.

I'm about five minutes from going on and sure enough I get kicked out of the meeting. Of course, I didn't get physically removed from a virtual room. My computer with the free trial of Skynet installed, sensing my distrust of technology, decided to increase my heartrate by lowering my bandwidth to a point to not be registered by the third-party hosting software or something technical like that. Well, played computer, you got me, now let me back in. I'm the speaker, the *speaker*! I run through the house yelling "get off the Wi-Fi!" dramatically, like I'm Matt Damon, then restart my computer and log back in, making it back with an embarrassing amount of time before they queue me in. I share my screen and bring up my bio, all without a hitch.

It's a strange new world we live in, focusing on a small circular dot above my computer screen, assuming there are people on the other side, but not knowing because of the lack of feedback I would normally be receiving if I were to be in "real time." I know that forty-eight people were present when I began my presentation, and barring a mass exodus once I went to "speaker mode," which is well within the scope of reality, there should still be a like number watching as I move from slide to slide. Still, I can't quite shake the feeling that I'm standing in my dining room talking to myself. Public speaking has never been an issue for me. I can get up in front of a room and talk about a bald spot on my testicles without trepidation or preparation. However, something I've found is that I have fear of standing for long periods of time in front of an audience, like some kind of ceremony. I just feel like I'm going to lock my legs and do one of those swaying pass-outs you see on funny videos.

They gave me twenty minutes of the meeting and I never like to use it all because invariably what I present will generate a question or two, and I want to allow time for that. I have done enough of these that I can adjust the slides and my pace to hit my time goal, which gives me great satisfaction, and after I answered a few questions, I closed my time by saying, "It's a crazy world out there, my friends.

Times are tough. Please take care of yourselves and take care of your people. If you or someone you know is in a dark place and needs to talk, I'm just a phone call away." It's always a relief when you finish and didn't do something or more importantly say something stupid that may lead to future anxiety. It feels even better when you are able to give someone an opportunity to talk, and they take you up on it and afterward feel better for doing it.

The presentation was the biggest thing on my schedule for today, and it's looking like a beautiful Friday afternoon where I'm left to my own devices. Back in my drinking days, I would hit the outdoor patio of a local taco shop and down as many margaritas as humanly possible, which would lead to a night of drinking and a following day of aspirin and regret. I'm not going to lie. There are times I miss the freedom of just doing something I wanted to do, not something I had to do, and other times I miss that feeling of freedom from giving a shit that inebriation brought.

I have no plans on wasting this afternoon on alcohol or work, so I checked my bike tires and decided to hit the local bike path for an afternoon mindfulness bike tour of the river. I know I've been all over, under, and around the whole mindfulness thing and how it helps me deal with my anxiety, but I recently got turned on to bringing mindfulness to more rote activities like walks or, in this case, rides. Its super easy to do and way more rewarding than I thought it would be. It begins like other sessions, breathing and steadying my mind before actually starting out, then it's just a question of riding my bike while being keenly aware of what I am feeling and taking in the whole of my experience, seeing the things that would normally escape my attention, appreciating to the fullest what I would normally take for granted. It was a cool experience, one I highly recommend, and it did wonders for my overall mood, I didn't even feel like yelling at the meth monkeys who camp out and make the riverbanks look like a dumpster exploded, at a ska music festival.

Upon my return home, I put my bike away and started a pot of coffee brewing. When it's hot and ready, Lisa and I will sit out on our back patio, in our authentic plastic Adirondack chairs, and go over the highs and lows while the dogs play musical laps to irritation.

I feel good about the day. I put myself out there professionally and personally regarding my depression. Time will tell if anyone wants to talk about either, but rest assured when they do, I will be willing, ready, and able.

SATURDAY, JULY 18, 2020

I had a much better night of sleep last night, I don't know why, and it's frustrating, not the sleep, but the not knowing, because whatever I did, I want to do it again. Who knows, it may have been my mindfulness bike ride yesterday afternoon, but I had some very pleasant dreams, which was a welcome change from the nightmare style, well, nightmares that have been more common in my life since my mental setback. I remember a dream where I was a squirrel, living in a house made of those thick specialty noodles you pay more for, and that I played the kazoo in a band consisting of three other squirrels a rabbit and Jack Black, and that we were all tired of his upstaging bullshit. I will tell you that when you haven't been sleeping so good, an extra hour of sleep is like a fresh twenty-dollar bill in an unexpected birthday card.

I got up, made the bed, did a workout, and was headed to the grocery store with Noah when my phone vibrated in my pocket. I can tell it's a text and not a call, but I'm far too conscientious a driver to check my phone while driving. Plus it's is in the side pockets of my cargo shorts that are secured with actual buttons and not Velcro, which makes it difficult to get to in a pinch. It was my friend Michelle asking if I had time to do a painting to put in a bare spot in their living room. I bet you didn't know that I was also an artist, though I use that term so loosely, it's falling off, and always with a chuckle. I'm an artist like Joel Osteen is a humble man of God, an argument could be made, but who am I kidding?

I learned early on in dealing with my depression the value that art and art therapy can bring to the situation. When I was thirteen and besieged by the infancy of my depression, I found that I could push away some of the debilitating effects by just sitting and doodling with a pen and paper. It was mostly just drawings of dicks and boobs, but the thesis was valid. When I was a little older, I watched this crazy German man on the Lawrence Welk channel paint an entire landscape painting in like twenty-some minutes. He would yell at the painting as he took his big brush, loaded it with gobs of paint, and then smashed it into the canvas like he was trying to kill a spider while on a carnival ride.

I was captivated and wanted more, which I got when I watched a gentler, far hairier man paint the same way, amazing landscapes in thirty minutes or less, guaranteed. His name was Bob Ross, and he would be an inspiration for me both artistically and psychologically, as I found that you could choose to see glaring fucking mistakes as happy accidents and carry small woodland creatures in your shirt pockets. I took what money I could scrape together and bought the lowest-quality dollar-store art supplies I could find. The brushes fell apart as they were being taken out of the package, the paint containers were half-dried, and the canvases were made of paper. I created with those meager implements the most sinister, grotesque, evil hellscapes you would ever experience. It was like Dante's *Inferno* but for adults. Unfortunately, I was trying to paint a peaceful mountain and happy little cabin.

As horrible as that first attempt was, it totally did the trick as far as my depression goes. The dark grasp of depression was held largely at bay by an activity, I had a real, useful tool, a tool that created abominations but still, a tool. As time passed, I began painting as an outlet, as a therapy and, I found, for enjoyment. As with any good thing there can be a dark side or be taken too far. I remember wanting to give a memorable gift and thinking to myself, "What could be a better gift than the greatest painting ever painted, by a painter."

My excitement built as I sprung for the slightly better grade of materials and developed the composition in my head, it was going to be amazing. I ran the conceptual motion picture over and over in my mind of when the magical gift was opened. As the wrapping paper was torn away, a bright light appeared as the sound of a chorus of angels could be heard in the periphery. Tears of joy streamed down the recipient's face and amazed wonder of the technical skill and craftsmanship. The only question that would linger would be which museum it should hang in first, probably the Smithsonian. All that was technically left to do was paint the damn thing and revel in the glory. You can probably imagine what happened. It was the Sony Betamax of paintings, the New Coke of paintings. It would have put Dwayne Johnson off eating protein. It went wrong from the beginning, then took a turn for the wrong-er, I would have been better served dipping marmots in paint and making them fight to the death on a canvas.

My vision of triumph and happiness had turned to terror. My plan had gone to shit and any money I had to buy a proper gift was spent on the upgraded supplies to create "An Ode to Satan's Hemorrhoids." I felt that art had betrayed me, that I had been abandoned by any degree of ability or talent, and that the tool I had grown so attached to, that had helped me through many battles, had suddenly disappeared, and I was scared. It led to a very hopeless time in my life that sucked, hard, but was valuable in my development as a survivor. I learned a priceless lesson through that period and that is "I can fuck up anything." I know what you're thinking, that I was just feeling sorry for myself and being a whiny little bitch. No, I realize you're not the kind of person that would call me a little bitch. I threw that in there for effect, sorry. What I meant by "I can fuck up anything" is that no matter how easy the task, no matter how many times I've successfully accomplished it before, if I put undue pressure on myself, or create grand expectations to live up to that, I can, literally, fuck anything up. So the lesson was to take it easy, do the best I can, and enjoy the process, then even if I do fuck up, I still received a benefit for doing it.

Through the years I've done a bunch of paintings, even a couple of murals, which wasn't as much fun as you might think because of the height that I had to work from. For most people, being on a sky-lift twenty feet in the air is not a problem; it would be "fun." I would get up there, and it would start swaying in the breeze, and I thought that I was going to fall and die, or more likely sprain an ankle, but the fact remains I don't like heights and sometimes depths. I've done a lot of spray paint art, mostly stencil work since my freestyle sucks. I've carved a little, sculpted a little, and done some block printing. Basically, if the project could make a mess around the house, I would be like "sold," Lisa would give me the stink-eye, and I would respond to her nonverbal intimidation by assuring her that I would clean it up thoroughly and to her standards. She would give me the "proceed at your own peril" nod, and I would get to work.

I believe in art therapy so much that I wanted to be involved in promoting it and introducing it to fellow sufferers. I mean you sit down do art, then feel better, easy-peasy, soft and cheesy. What I found however is that art therapy is an actual thing. It requires board certifications and licenses and shit. I would have to go through classes and pay for those classes. So I did what any self-respecting, unlicensed, back-alley art pusher would do. I spent a bunch of money I didn't have to rent an upstairs room at a crappy little strip mall, and I went ahead and did it anyway. I got some cheap foldout tables and uncomfortable metal folding chairs. I brought all my excess art supplies and bought a bunch of stuff at the dollar store. I was committed to introducing art to people suffering with depression and wasn't going to let anything stop me including the fact that I couldn't do it, and thus the Blue Funk Society was born.

I called it the Blue Funk Society as a sarcastic commentary on the belief held by some nonsufferers that how we feel is somehow a choice, that instead of experiencing depression, we are just 'feeling blue" or are in a "mood" or "funk." The question is, can something you say be sarcastic if you're the only one who knows what you're talking about? The answer is "Who cares." People liked the name, which irritated me slightly, but as it turned out, the Blue Funk Society was probably the dumbest, most awesome thing I have ever tried. I say that it was dumb solely due to the fact that there was no viable business plan whatsoever, no way to capture revenue or offset operational expenditures. The original plan was to charge a per visit fee or a monthly membership, but I was really bad at asking for money, and many depressed people are depressed because they have no money. It was like me opening up a Subway sandwich shop, putting in ovens and work stations, various meats and cheeses and vegetables, putting in seats and tables and napkin dispensers, everything you could think of, except for a cash register.

In the over four months of operating the Blue Funk Society, I was out over fifteen hundo per month while bringing in an average of forty-two dollars per month. That being said, it was awesome. I would prepare small canvases with a basic drawing for everyone, and as people would arrive, we would begin the same painting together. It was like a painting party, without the party. What we did is simply paint and talk, we wouldn't talk about heavy deep personal issues while painting, The idea was that if you could talk about anything, you could talk about everything, so if I could get someone to just join into a conversation about the local sports team while engaging in a group activity, that it would be easier for them to talk to their professional about how they feel. I didn't offer advice and in no way held myself out as someone with knowledge or authority. I was simply facilitating a meeting, but word had started to get out about this unsanctioned paint club with only one rule, so the heat was on. I was fielding more and more calls wanting to know my reasoning and methodology, and since I had neither coupled with no revenue, I decided that this little experiment had run its course.

I always thought about bringing it back, but this time doing it legit, getting an old Winnebago, gutting it, putting the tables and chairs inside, and then driving to remote locations where I could conduct cheap painting sessions without the "art fuzz" ever knowing or having the ability to track me down. Of course, I don't know how I would find the people, and once found, how I would get them to pay me, but businesses have started with worse ideas. Look at Kenny Rogers Roasters.

There is no doubt that art and depression have a long history together. Most people would look at it from the point of view of the depression, rather than the art, conjuring images of Vincent van Gogh or Ludwig van Beethoven masters whose work could only be overshadowed by the impact depression played in their lives. The same could be said for Edvard Munch, Francisco Goya, and Georgia O'Keeffe. We're they and countless others depressed because their minds were wired more for creativity, or did the creativity develop because of their depression? I know that science has by now figured it out to the genomic sequence that occurs right after conception, but I have never really bought into that. I think that there is a very fine line between brilliance and madness, and that the closer a person gets to one, the closer they get to both.

Anyway, I am far more concerned with art not as it relates to depression but rather how art can be used as a treatment. Again, I'm not a professional in any way, I don't profess to have anything but firsthand personal knowledge and belief. There have literally been thousands of studies done in this area, covering every conceivable angle, so I'm going to let you open your magic Google box and go nuts. What I will say, and again, you can look it up, is that brain scans have been done on a depressed person before and after they have engaged in art therapy, and the results are nothing short of amazing. In the example that I saw, the "before" image showed very little of the brain activity or engagement, whereas the "after" scan showed vast areas in color, meaning that the therapy resonated across much of the brain.

As of right now, there is no "cure" for depression, only varied treatment options. Sitting down, making a mess, and doing something creative will not make depression go away forever, but it will offer a degree of respite and shelter from a raging storm that I highly encourage you to take advantage of. When you do sit down for "craft time," a couple of things will help maximize the positivity. Don't expect to be good at something if you've never done it. Be present and enjoy the experience without adding expectations on yourself. Don't overthink it. When you were a kid at school and the teacher said that it was craft time, did you plan an elaborate composition with correct perspective and fixed source of light, did you microman-age the materials and supplies, or did you just jump in make a mess and have fun? I don't exactly know at what point in our development we lose the ability to just be free and fun and spontaneous, but revert, I say, revert to your inner child once in a while. Once you've begun all you have to do is not forget to breathe and smile. It's okay to have a little fun. Fuck your depression.

SUNDAY, JULY 19, 2020

A two-part question to start the day. Do you have a porch, and if not, do you ever wish you had a porch? I'm talking about a proper porch that you could have a good sit on a summer Sunday morning, steam rising from your freshly poured mug of coffee, non-crows happily chirping away in the freshness of a new day. If I had a porch, then I could also have one of those wood-framed screen doors that would close with a "clap" as it contacted the wooden doorjamb. I can't imagine that I wouldn't have a nice old rocking chair or hanging bench seat, just to show off the luxurious girth of the wood plank floor. Of course, there would be a round wicker table, the perfect size for holding a carafe of coffee in the morning, and all the fixings, but equally at ease holding a pitcher of iced tea or lemonade in the afternoon.

I don't have a porch. I have a three-foot-wide covered concrete slab walkway that leads to a nondescript wood entry door guarded by a metal storm door that hasn't had a handle on it in eleven years. Hang on, now all of a sudden that fact is starting to bother me. Where did the handle go? I have no idea whatsoever where the handle is. What happened to it, and probably most apropos, why haven't I put a new handle on? Regardless, I don't have a porch, and upon reflection, I have never lived in a house with a proper porch, and I'm old. What I do have is a crappy back patio, so I will take my porch envy and my cup of earthy, full-bodied bean bliss outside where I will sit in my genuine plastic Adirondack chair, take a sip, ignore the crows and their ceaseless ca-cawing, rest my head back on the plastic slats, close my eyes, and enjoy the moment.

Later today, Lisa and I will get out of the house and maybe hike to a waterfall, or maybe I'll pump up our inflatable raft and do a quick river float. We haven't decided on what exactly, but there will be fresh air and sunshine. I have learned some interesting things lately about myself in doing the meditation and contemplation. I realize that in summers before that I would have small regrets when not being able to make the most of summer. I think that I mentioned that to you at some point earlier. What I found out was that I actually purposefully sabotaged a great deal of the summer not because I couldn't figure out what to do or because time was lost in the planning, but because I didn't feel good about myself and didn't really want to do anything, but mostly I didn't want to feel guilty about not doing anything. I know that on the major breakthrough scale this little nugget is more toward the "meh" side of the scale, but it's still useful information that can be applied to managing the "me" of today. So now we're just going to load up head out and go do something that will make today enjoyable, especially given the topic I've chosen to discuss. Finally, it's suicide day, yay. The yay was dripping with sarcasm, in case you missed it.

There can be no open unabridged discussion about depression without including suicide as a talking point. I will not apologize for wanting to talk about a subject that nobody seems to want to talk about. By understanding more about where people are and what makes them do what they do, perhaps we can help people and keep them with us longer, so we need more and more frank, unapologetic discussions about suicide. Keep in mind, as we walk down this path, that I am very bad at suicide, always have been, and hopefully I can continue to be until the dinosaurs come back and eat us all, making suicide a moot point. What makes me confident that I am qualified to talk on this subject is the fact that for years I have fantasized about suicide, have planned it, and have desperately wanted it to happen so much that I have begun my attempt many times. I've sat for hours staring down the barrel of a loaded gun, finger on the trigger, just waiting for the release that millisecond of action would bring. So yes, my friend, I know suicide all too well, and that's not something anyone should have to say.

It's no coincidence that I'm bringing this subject up to you on a Sunday. Together with its pal Monday, they make up the two most popular days of the week people choose to take their lives, and if you're curious about what is the most popular day of the year, when most suicides occur, it's New Year's Day. If you've connected the dots between the two, you realize that there is a link. They both represent something that people with depression despise, a beginning. The start of a new week or the start of a new year can be devastating to someone who just wants the pain to stop, who feel like they can't exist within the dark anguish of their depression and that enduring for long would fall into the realm of the impossible.

Let me say this to you: if you have thought about taking your life, or maybe you've even planned it a little, don't freak out; you're not alone or crazy. A bigger cross-section of the population has been where you are than you could imagine; it is our nature to explore all our options when going through difficult times. Seek help, find a friend to talk to, find an enemy to talk to, and take control. If you are tired of carrying your burden and the thought of starting another week makes you want to, well, kill yourself, follow the following instructions exactly. Empty your hands. Hold your right hand flat away from your body at shoulder height, palm facing upward. Pick an object directly in your sight line and focus on it. Now move that right hand quickly toward your exposed cheek until it makes contact, hopefully with an audible noise. That is from me to you. The world is better with you in it. Asshole! You are here for a purpose, and while you may not believe that or have felt it yet, it's true. It might be that you're here to keep another asshole from killing themselves. Now call 1-800-273-8255 and do fucking everything they tell you to do.

I'm going to talk about my experiences with suicide, and I may use humor. I don't know any other way, but know this, there is nothing funny or honorable about suicide; it's depression winning, and I fucking hate when that fucking fucker wins. My job, your job, every person's job is to not allow that to happen. Depression will achieve the upper hand from time to time, may even win a battle or two, but it must be defeated at all costs when it comes to your life. Everyone got that? Good.

I first thought about suicide, seriously, when I was in my late twenties. I think that it goes without saying that my ideations of ending it all coincided with my darkest of days. Why do people say that it goes without saying, and then say it anyway? Regardless, I didn't have a specific reason that I wanted to commit suicide other than the darkness, anguish, and pain that I wanted to stop, I hadn't experienced abuse, or lost an irreplaceable love, or committed an act that I couldn't accept forgiveness for, just ceaseless, tormenting unhappiness that permeated every fiber of my being. As permanent and never-ending as it felt at the time, it turns out that the intensity was only transitory and that I was able, with maximum effort, to pull out of the dive and go on with life. I was wrong and I wholeheartedly and freely admit it. I thought the intense pain would last forever, and it almost did. If there is a moral to this story it's to never solve a temporary problem with a permanent solution, you're only going to pass your pain on to someone you love. I was wrong; it got better.

Reasons aside, for me suicide was a foregone conclusion, I was going to do it, it was just a matter of "how." You see, while I wanted my pain and suffering to be over, I didn't want the endeavor to actually hurt or to physically make me suffer. I know, call me a total pussy if you want, but people survive suicide attempts all the time and are forced to live in abject corporeal misery until their dying breath. It is possible to tackle a moving freight train and not be killed, people have shot themselves in the face and have not died, and there are those who have leapt from the Golden Gate Bridge and are amazingly around to tell the tale. There is so much to consider when planning your death—angles and effectiveness, chance and circumstance, and the inevitability of the unforeseen consequences.

If someone at the spur of the moment just up and kills themselves successfully, there is likelihood in my opinion that it was an accident, a mistake, or they had spent so much time in the "death zone" that desperation overtook them. I say that because my experience with suicide and suicidal people has led me to form the conclusion that most suicidal people don't want to die. They want the pain to die, the sorrow they feel to die. They want the burden they carry to be lifted from their shoulders. Real suicides aren't a cowardly person's last desperate act to evade punishment for committing a heinous crime. Real suicides take thought and planning, sweating all the intricate details, including a suicide note and who will find your body.

I bought a special bullet when I was thinking that my end would come via self-inflicted gunshot wound. It was a Federal Hydra-Shok nine-millimeter round that, given my gun's barrel length, would exit the muzzle at around twelve hundred feet per second and, with its hollow-point design, would expand upon first impact, creating a much bigger exit hole going out than the one coming in. It would do the job admirably, and I only needed one, but they made me buy the whole box, which was expensive. I decided to hold the gun at a seventy-five-degree angle under my chin, with the front sight resting directly above my Adam's apple. Holding it in my mouth or to my temple had too many negative outcomes, meaning people lived. Keep in mind that your calculations have to account for a shaky hand. The closer I got to pulling the trigger, the more my hand would shake.

As planned, I drove to a secluded spot, down by the river, off the beaten path, but not too far. I would sit alone, allowing my commitment to solidify into action. My handwriting is illegible to even me, so my suicide note was word processed and printed. I wanted my feelings known and not misunderstood. I signed it formally, as I have done so many business letters in my life, but this one broke my heart completely. I folded the letter sharply and sealed it in an envelope with "Lisa" as the only hint as to the recipient. I sat the letter in the absolute center of the passenger seat and adjusted my body in such a way that the bullet. Once it exited my skull, it would lodge in the frame of the car and not have enough energy to hurt anyone else. The gunshot would probably be heard by somebody, but my body would most likely be discovered the following morning by an early runner or dog walker. I imagined the shock and sadness felt by my family and friends, but it would pass, and they would indeed be better off. I felt the front sight dig in to my skin as I rested the gun in place and mentally checked the angles. I closed my eyes and put my finger on the trigger. I applied a little pressure and could feel the composite trigger move against the gun body. This was it. Like I said, I'm not the best at suicide. I couldn't ever commit that last two-inch pounds of force required, and for that I'm exceedingly grateful.

Those days were the fucking worst. I remember each time like it was yesterday, remember what I was wearing, remember putting the gun down after making it safe, not sure if I was relieved or disappointed. It was like that feeling of opening homemade jam, it could be the sweet strawberry that my mom had perfected over the years, or it could be the fucking blackberry where you're picking seeds out of your teeth for three days. I was still adrift on the ocean with no oars. The only communication was the nonstop screaming in my head from my depression telling me that I couldn't even kill myself correctly. It was the absolute worst, but I kept living and kept working and things got better. Over the years I went through many difficult periods where suicide moved continuously up the list of feasible options. Each time that I would give it serious thought, there was a part of my brain that would shoot the idea down or immediately discount it.

"What about a hose running from the exhaust to the inside of the car?" You need a goddamn garage to pull that one of genius. You just can't sit in your driveway while the world walks their dogs by and waves. "What about all those old meds? Take a handful, wash it down with vodka, go to bed, and never wake up. Would that work?" No, I would just end up with vomit all over my face and a hangover, no thanks. "Slit the wrists in a warm bath and just slide into oblivion?" Blood is gross and sticky, and it will get all over me and imagine the mess, if I did that I'd better die, or Lisa would kill me and void the whole process. "Why don't you just hang yourself?" What am I, in prison?

Truth be told, there were three moments that my life hung by a thread, and another time that I was closer to the brink than I should have been. Each time I battled back to regain my rightful place as a functioning, taxpaying citizen. After each occasion came periods of absolute joy and wonder, experiences that I would have robbed myself of. I've gained knowledge and understanding that I could never have passed to anyone, and now because I still live, I get to go on the offensive. I get to take the fight to my depression. I don't know where you are right now. We may have covered much of the same ground, you and I, in our struggles, so I'm not going to give you some bullshit motivation like "just hang in there," even though you should just hang in there. The deal is that life isn't fair; it never has been. You feel it, many of your important questions will go unanswered, and often justice and acceptance will feel just out of reach, and you will make a choice. Know this, we need you in this fight. We need your voice, your experience. If you give up, if you give in, that will remain your legacy forever. However, if you fight on, then through, and because of that struggle are able to reach out your hand and help one person, then you are a warrior, a hero, a veteran of the silent war, displaying strength and honor where you once felt weakness.

Depression wants you dead. It craves the abyss and gains strength the closer you are to the edge. It sells you soul darkness and despair. It voids all scraps of hope that don't serve its shadowy purposes and tells you that you are powerless to challenge its dominion over you. Unless you are among the boldest, most dedicated to ending your suffering, then there may just be a means for you to break free. Depression delights as you sow the seeds of your own destruction, and it fertilizes those seeds by fueling your resolve and waters them by negating any other viable option. Depression plays you like a cheesy cardboard recorder. It knows you, knows your strengths and weaknesses, and knows what you want more than anything. It's like when you talk about something, then it suddenly pops up on your timeline, especially if it's something that you could use to actually kill yourself with.

Listen, there are many reasons why people kill themselves, and I don't claim to know how they all feel or that I have an answer. What I will say is that it's not killing yourself. I can't imagine a situation that couldn't be made better by living, even if in the end it's just to tell others that dying is no way live a life. If you're lonely, fight on. If you're in pain, fight on. If you feel bullied and that it will never get better, fight on. If you've lost your money and status, fight on. If you've hurt someone and can't live with it, fight on. If you've lost faith and hope, fight on. If all you have in your fucking life is the fucking fight and you're fucking tired and want to fucking rest, *fight fucking on*!

Seek help my friends and then accept help, make each day above ground a victory, mark it down on your calendar, and show it to your depression. Do something you never do, go jump in the ocean, then make sure you get out, see how much ice cream you could fit in your mouth, go see a movie and invite someone you haven't seen in a while, then smile, goddammit, *smile*. Take your life back one step away from the brink at a time.

I learned something recently and have meditated on it, so I would like to share it with you, and I think that this would be the perfect venue for that. I want to talk to you about being broken. Broken people commit suicide, broken people think about and plan suicide, and broken people feel no hope. I was a broken person. The world broke me, and depression seized upon that brokenness, giving me no purpose other than to complete my dark destiny of becoming dump fodder. When we experience this, we believe that there is no way that we will ever be useable never be able to fulfill any purpose.

I want to talk to you about kintsugi, something that on the surface has nothing to do with depression or suicide, but bear with me please. Kintsugi is a Japanese art form of repairing broken or damaged pottery by using gold and silver metal powder, mixed with lacquer. In Japan, kintsugi transcends art to become a philosophy that treats breakage and repair as the history of an object to be celebrated, not disguised or discarded. There are shattered pieces, devoid of use or worth that are completely reconditioned to beautiful, operational whole items but done in such a way that the item's past and all that it has experienced is emphasized and adds significance to the repair.

We all need to embrace this amazing philosophy and understand that if it could be done with pottery, it can absolutely be done with you. You can be made whole and given a purpose. You will bear the scars of your struggles, of that there could be no doubt, but those scars will be a testament to your fortitude will be a beacon to others who feel broken and without worth and will allow you and those around you to remember where you came from and celebrate where you are going. Being broken is often less a choice and more a result

of circumstance, diagnosis, and misfortune. Staying broke is undeniably a choice, but this isn't a Disney movie. The pottery doesn't
come to life at night and kintsugi itself back together while singing
"Cracked and Shellacked," then magically appear whole and complete as the sun rises over Mt. Fuji. I don't actually know if it would
rise or set over Mt. Fuji. I've never been to Japan because I don't like
eating fish, and yes, I know that shellac and lacquer are different, but
try rhyming with *lacquer*; it's not easy.

Nevertheless, it takes a kintsugi master a long time, hard work,
and attention to the smallest detail to deftly repair the structural
integrity of a broken piece of pottery, just as it will take someone
versed in restoring people to their former glory to move a person
from a broken state, to a healthy purposeful human being. If you feel
fragmented and don't know what to do, make a call, reach out to your
doctor or other healthcare provider, and be open and honest. Suicide
is not the answer, unless the question was "What's the goddamn stupidest fucking solution to a problem ever employed by humankind?"
Keep in mind that's coming from someone who almost did it, three
times. Listen carefully, I said this earlier, and I will restate in now for
emphasis—this fight needs you; we need your voice now more than
ever. Does that mean your pain will diminish? I can't tell you it will
or won't, but I will say that it will have a purpose behind it, and if I'm
living proof of anything, it's that life can and will get better, if you
give yourself the chance.

MONDAY, JULY 20, 2020

Do you ever feel like sometimes you just might be losing your mind? I know that it's a slippery slope sometimes. This morning my eyes opened, I checked the time and realized it was Monday, that it's still 2020, and that I might be losing my mind. I had a dream that some "patriot" shot me in the dick because I was wearing a mask to protect my fellow man that made me look like Margaret Thatcher. I don't know what offended the gunslinging, Bible-thumping, camo-wearing flag waver more, the fact that I was wearing a mask to help flatten the curve, or that I looked like a former British prime minister. The part that I find most bizarre is that if I saw that story on the nightly news, I would totally believe it.

It's Monday, or should I say Mon-yay? Today I'm going to start something that I've been meditating about. I know that I mentioned to you yesterday that Monday is one of the days of the week that people choose to commit suicide or suicide attempts. Mondays and depression go together like politics and loss of smell, but what if, for just one day, I just don't say the word "have," instead replacing it with the word "get," that's all, just being mindful on one word. By doing so I no longer *have* to go to work; I *get* to go to work. I don't *have* to do chores around the house, pay bills, or have to do anything. I'm *blessed* to have a job, to have a house, even if it means there will be chores and bills. I'm *blessed* to be physically and mentally able to do stuff. It's amazing the change that one word can make in your life and outlook.

For so long Monday has been more an enemy to conquer, obstacle to overcome than an actual day in my life. But you realize there

202

are only so many sunrises and that not making the most of every single one is an appalling waste. So now I *get* to take this pack of hyena-huahuas around the savanna so they can dine on human ankle flesh. I will say as I get older, I appreciate personal growth more and more. It's not always fun, it's often painful and embarrassing, but if you're not doing, learning, and growing, then you are missing out on achieving your maximum potential. So many times, people suffering with depression get bogged down in the fight that there is absolutely no point in self-improvement. It's like a frontline soldier taking a correspondence course to become an actuary while actively taking fire. I could actually gauge how deep down the rabbit hole I was by determining how concerned I was about the future. The healthier the level, the more I would do to positively affect my personal and business outlook, like working out or engaging in activities to promote my business.

We need to work together to flip that script. We need to find those who are currently in the trenches, fighting hand to hand, and give them something else to do, something to focus on. Let me tell you that if I can get a win, any win during a time of tribulation, it's like a shot of Vitamin B_{12} and Red Bull right to the veins, like when you're at the gym and just want to stop, but then AC/DC comes on, and you're right back in it, baby! By far the biggest problem that people who suffer from depression have, besides the depression, is "fuck it." There is an overwhelming desire when confronted with a difficulty or responsibility during times of struggle to just say "fuck it," and either ignore it or treat it with contempt. This is obviously a big deal when you're talking about important things like personal and business relationships, communication, and finances.

I'm going to talk about finances for a minute, then I'll bring it right back around to how we're going to deal with "fuck it," so bear with me a minute. Money has always been an issue for me, always been one of my major stressors, and often one of my depression's best friends. I know what you're thinking, Judgy McJudgerson, that I'm in the financial services industry and should know all about and have a complete handle on personal finances. Knowing something and living it are two separately unequal entities. I run a business that more mouths than mine depend on, and when you're in that position, what you make isn't what you bring home and money is always tighter than you want it to be. When you factor in the added expense that raising differently abled children often requires, on top of the major expenses that life throws at you to keep things interesting, like having to buy new tires, washing machine, or luxury Frisbees, then money can be a real dick punch, right to the dick.

Money is the leading cause of stress in America today, and for many people the only exercise they have done during COVID-19 is running out of it. It seems like you can't stand on your front porch and throw a burning alcohol bottle into a crowd of antifascists without catching at least three people who are unemployed on fire. I should probably say that I would never actually catch someone on fire, even antifascists, who may be against fascism, but are totally into being dicks. Money is such a wide-ranging topic that I could spend hours and hours just rubbing it all over my body, letting each bill in the stack flutter erotically to the floor, so I will limit the scope to money and depression.

Let's get this out of the way. First, money, or more specifically the lack of it, is not a cause of clinical depression. You may look at your bank account or in your wallet and feel sadness or stress, or a combination of both, but being poor doesn't cause depression like being rich doesn't cure it. That being said, for those of us who do suffer, our depression loves money and the hardships that it can bring to our lives psychologically. If you're thinking about killing yourself because of money, you're not even making the depression work for it. It's like when the NBA players were allowed to be on team USA in the Olympics. Just give them the fucking gold medal when they get off the plane and spare us from watching crappy lopsided basketball. The problem is that we tie ourselves to money on many levels, our ego, our self-image, our personal well-being, even our happiness in one way or the other is tied to money. We measure success not in our good works or how many people we helped, but it what we got paid for it, what kind of car we drive, if we have natural stone countertops or belong to a country club.

The way to deal with it, from a sufferer's point of view, is to devalue it, to discount the value and power that it holds over you emotionally. But that is much easier said than done, and it's more deeply ingrained in human nature than you may believe. Humans and money problems started shortly after Adam and Eve received the great news that they were preapproved for a *golden* delicious MasterCard, with a low introductory APR. The Quran, the Torah, and the Bible all talk about money and the importance of not being an asshole in dealing with it. The Bible goes so far as to call it "the root of all evil," which is pretty heavy but completely understandable. When we are depressed, we long for anything that will distract us from our pain that will allow us to feel something, anything, so we go online and buy something. Now we feel excitement and anticipation waiting for that thing to arrive. Once it does, we feel happiness, albeit artificial, but still it feels better than what we were feeling. When the feeling wears off, or when we receive the bill, we feel worse, which adds to our depression, which makes us long for anything that will distract us, and so on and so forth.

So we have this huge chunk our self-image tied to money, and we have this colossal desire to buy happiness, and then, on top of that, we need stuff to survive, like food, medicine, shelter, clothes, and toilet paper, unless you've become on old-timey fur trader, they all still require someone to get paid. I'm never going to get on my soapbox and tell you that money isn't important, or that you should shun worldly possessions and go live in the woods in a hollowed-out tree trunk where you have a pet raccoon named Colonel Shifty and make your clothes out of woven pine needles and tree sap. What I will tell you is that I understand where you are. I have been there myself, and there are some things you can work on that won't fully devalue the effect of money on your life but will keep it more manageable and in perspective.

First of all, understand that by being a depressed person you deal with a set of circumstances others may not have to, and you need to be cognizant and honest about the power it holds over you. When you are deeply affected, such as experiencing mania or are at a level of "fuck it," your success or failure will be solely reliant on "damage control." Sometimes the best thing you can do with your money is keep it in your wallet. Get rid of your credit cards, don't keep them with you, especially in unstable times, and replace them instead with a prepaid card that has a set amount loaded. You may wake up the next day having spent more than you wanted, but not all you could have. Also, steer clear of your problem establishments, and don't act like you don't know what I'm talking about. I used to love buying drinks for people. I don't know why, maybe because they liked me more, and the more I bought, the more popular I became, which is sad and pathetic but mostly sad. Regardless, you know that place, whether it's actual or virtual, that magically makes money uncontrollably fly out of your wallet or purse. Limit your exposure until you are feeling stronger.

The next piece of advice has been around since day one but still remains valid and important—pay yourself first. Pay your rent or mortgage, pay your utility company, buy groceries and all necessities first and without hesitation, then feel good about it and tell yourself that what you did was important and appreciated. If you are lucky enough to have a few dollars left after responsibility took its cut, then by all means, indulge yourself; buy that bacon-scented candle, taco sleeping bag, or genuine alpaca panties and feel good. Just don't over indulge or use credit cards, because that will just add to your responsibilities next month. I'm going to take a moment and talk about credit cards because it seems like I'm dissing on them, and I don't want to be misunderstood.

Credit cards are the absolute fucking worst things you could own, and that's coming from someone who's been involved with timeshares. They are not there to make your life easier or financially stable; they want you to buy shit you can't afford then make minimum payments that take forever to pay it off. Your life will be far better off mentally and financially if you steer well clear of all of them, my opinion, for what it's worth. What about keeping a credit card for emergencies? Good question, thanks for asking. I know for myself that if I have a card and I'm at or around "fuck it" as far as mindset and outlook, I'm not thinking about the future or an unforeseen emergency that may or may not ever happen. I will ride that bitch like a rented mule. Even if I feel "fuck it" coming on and do the right thing and hide the card or freeze it in a block of ice, those cocksuckers at the credit card companies will send out blank checks that you can use for anything, including cash. Listen, each individual has to make their own decisions based on their known behavior patterns, but even credit cards kept for a good reason can be an enemy.

Keep in mind that everything I talk about is based on my experience, I have made all the mistakes, done all the wrong things, for the sole express purpose of telling you what to do with your money. Believe me, I have seen the dark side. I have lost friends and clients because of money, seen grown people behave childishly. I have been robbed and lied to, and I've known of people who have gone to prison or killed themselves because of money. The best thing you can do is foster a healthy relationship with your money, and the easiest way to do that is to start saving it. I know that sounds stupid, but I get the same feeling when I'm able to save money that I used to get when I spent it and will often rather go without something I want if it means taking money out of savings to buy it. Saving money is healthy on several levels because it's your money, and next month, there will be more of it, and it's not something that can be held over your head or demanded of you, unless you are in fact being robbed, and in that case, choose safety.

Sometimes we, as depressed people, feel that we may cosmically be owed something for having to deal with all the bullshit and darkness. So when we feel "fuck it," there seems to be a justification for that behavior in the balancing of the scales, like we will be forgiven any trespasses that occurred while on a negative cycle of behavior, and frankly, nothing is farther from the truth, not even that coffee is made from beans, because it isn't; it's made from seeds that look like beans, so they were called beans. So if you're thinking that slack is being cut for you just because you have depression. Unless your mom's in charge, chances are, it's merely coincidental. You are now, and always, responsible for your actions no matter what level of depression you find yourself at, so if you get to "fuck it" and ride through your town naked on a demon unicorn burning every bridge you come across, your job, your family and friends, and your bank account know that you will have face the consequences.

Because what happens if you don't kill yourself? What happens when the sun comes up and, all of a sudden, you realize that you made it through the storm but your reputation didn't or some dear friendships didn't? How dark and stormy do those next clouds look on the horizon? I can't stop asking questions. Why? We have to know where we are my friends and take appropriate steps to limit the damage that will inevitably be done, not just financially but in all aspects of our lives, and it starts with communication.

Holy shit, stop the presses. Deevers is talking about talking again. It may be the last time he ever mentions it, so we better pay attention. Wow, that was pretty snarky even for me. If we don't tell people where we are emotionally or psychologically, they have no way of knowing where we are at, especially if you're a master thespian like many of us are. We perform the role that we want other people to see us as, so we don't have to talk, so we don't have to open up. It's a great system right up until it's not, and then the truth comes out and people are hurt, and we feel worse and the stigma of depression marches forward. If we talk to people, say, "I just wanted to let you know that I suffer from depression and do a pretty good job managing it, but if I appear to be acting erratically, or if I do or say something that's troubling, please bear with me as I work through it. Thank you."

You don't have to overthink it, you just talk about it; let people know. The more people who know the greater the support built up around you, the easier communication will be. People want to be part of a solution, by opening up to them you are bringing them into your life, you are presenting them with the problem, and you are allowing them to be a part of the solution. Then more people you have around you that know you and what you go through the easier it will be to say "I'm struggling, could you help me" or "Take my credit card and don't give it back until I feel better."

We need to focus on knowing where we're at and making ourselves better each and every day. We need to set ourselves up for victory when we start to struggle, not just wait for the defeat, and we do that by being proactive, by communicating by building that safety net that will be under us when we're on the high wire. Listen, there are no prizes handed out when your time is up on earth, I mean besides the heaven thing. You won't get a medal for having great credit or paying all your bills on time. I'm not saying you don't have to pay your bills. You do, every month, but money is an area that you have control over, so make wise decisions and work hard to take this weapon away from your depression.

TUESDAY, JULY 21, 2020

Good morning to you, my dear friend, I trust you slept well. I had one of those dark, turbulent nights where you receive visits from ghosts of past transgressions who want to teach you valuable lessons but you just want to drive your Zamboni to the petting zoo so you can feed the miniature goats. Then I had this dream that I ate one of my dogs. I don't know which one because they all look the same cooked, but I remember running out of Salsa Lizano, which is my favorite condiment hands down, imported directly from Costa Rica. Regardless, I was so upset that we were out that I didn't eat the dog. Instead, I threw it to my pet marshmallow, Fluffy, who apparently is carnivorous, and enjoyed eating one of my dogs because of some pet rivalry dynamic. Dreams are like weird little foreign films, written by Dr. Seuss, directed by Quentin Tarantino, with special effects by the Claymation people who did the raisin thing. Needless to say, I was happy to wake up.

Since I was happy to be alive after a harrowing night, that first cup of coffee tasted like the warm smile of an old friend too long removed and victory. It was rich and bold and hot and the perfect balance of goodwill and harmony that made me want to find a cottage and curl up next to the fire. However, it's Tuesday and that means we just can't sit around our imaginary cottage curled up next to our imaginary fire, no, we have real shit that needs to be done today, we have a meeting at the office with a client later, emails to compose and stuff to be filed and uploaded, and my shirts still dry, meaning a workout is also a something we need to do, so we should start moving with some purpose. And I know I said a gaggle of "wes" there, but I was mostly talking about me, so don't freak out.

I'm going to get moving on this stuff, but I also need to start looking at my upcoming therapy session with Dr. K in like two days. These last couple of weeks just flew by, and I still feel super optimistic about the direction that I'm heading, which feels like every day is a new record for most consecutive days of positive thinking and action, which is good, but also a little scary because I don't want it to stop because I don't want to experience a reversing trend in my thoughts or behaviors. I think it would be a good time to talk about exactly where I am right now as it relates to my depression and overall outlook. I experience depression every day. I literally do not remember the last depression-free day that I experienced in my life. Obviously if I would have known at the time, I would have made a bigger deal about it, maybe ate a cake. It was back when I used to eat cake.

It will happen like the bills will find their way to my mailbox, like my money will find its way out of my paycheck before it rests in my hands. It will visit, just like it always does. Now before we start composing sad songs with harps and shit about how everything sucks. I think it's important for you to know that while I deal with depression on the daily. The impact that it has on my life varies greatly. While I feel it, lately I have been able to move beyond its grasp and work on myself, and get work done, and feel good and look forward to things like therapy appointments. My headspace is good and positive, and I really feel like I may have turned a corner in my existence with depression, and that's not the depression or one of its derivative manias talking. I'm going to say something that I've said before. I think on more than one occasion, but nobody paid attention, probably because I was talking a lot of shit at the time, and it got lost in the noise, but it's possible for a person to be depressed and happy at the same time. Did you just say bullshit? No, really, it's true, I've experienced it myself and more recently than you may believe.

I think we first need to talk about happiness, which, besides genital herpes, is a depressed person's favorite topic of conversation. We just love talking about being happy. We need to refine its overarching parameters and nebulous nature for the purposes of this discussion, so when I talk about happiness, it will relate to one of two factors about the experience. The first factor is a current experience, or a feeling or emotion that makes you feel a fleeting sensation of happiness. The second factor is more an appraisal of a long-term satisfaction about life, about general, long-term quality of life. Both of these factors represent happiness on different timelines, and each can play a part toward the other. Let me give you an example. My beautiful, glorious cup of coffee made me happy this morning. It was a transitory sensation that by itself wouldn't give my life greater meaning, but experiencing that feeling no matter how temporarily, regularly over a period of time, can lead to feelings of greater life satisfaction. Now, conversely if I tell you that I have been loving my coffee since I switched to the organic fair-trade acorn milk creamer, then what are the chances, given I still have creamer, that I will love the next cup of coffee and that it too will make me happy? I would say the answer is pretty good, about the chances.

Let's dive just a little deeper about this happiness stuff before we jump to our conclusions. So we have ephemeral happiness and enduring happiness, and each can play in the others sandbox, to a degree. For the scope of our discussion I believe that it's important to recognize where happiness comes from, or at least a theory of how it develops and manifests itself in a person's life. Don't cite anything I'm about to tell you as actual fact. At this point together you should just damn know that I'm in no position to hold anything up as a factual representation. What I say should be treated like a political advertisement paid by Vladimir Putin, starring Pastor Peter Popoff. Now that I've given you my standard disclaimer, let's talk about Maslow's hierarchy of needs, and no, I didn't just make that up.

Maslow's hierarchy of needs is something I learned about back in college that has always stuck with me because of my depression and because it agrees with my overall thesis, or I would have discarded it with all the other Freudian prattle. Maslow's hierarchy is a pyramid scheme where the person above you takes all of your money and is happier, the end. Just kidding, that's elementary school recess. Imagine the Great Pyramid of Giza. Now picture the first few courses of stones, these are the widest as they are the foundation of the entire structure. In Maslow's Hierarchy this level represents our physiological needs: air, food, water, shelter and clothing, the bare essentials to sustain life. The next couple of courses of our great pyramid is narrower and represents our safety needs, such as physical security, our job, available resources and property, and protecting ourselves and our way of life. As we climb higher and narrower, we reach love and belonging, which includes friendship, intimacy, family, and a connection with community. Right after love we reach esteem level, narrower still, but this level represents respect, self-esteem, status, recognition, strength, and freedom. Finally, we have reached the apex of our pyramid; this level is self-actualization and is all about being the ultimate best version of yourself possible.

Okay, now you have Maslow's hierarchy of needs in graphical format in your head. The base of the pyramid is just that, our basic needs, and as you work through the narrowing sections, the focus changes dramatically from the real and the tangible to the ethereal but no less important aspects of life. My query to you is simply this: given what I just talked about, where does happiness come from? Or more to the point, how does it fit it with this example? Don't worry, there is not going to be homework assigned. Let's work through it together as kind of a bonding activity.

The question is, given there is both long- and short-term happiness, would you find either in the first level, or more to the point, if you just had air, food, water, shelter, and clothes, could you be happy? In my opinion, you could absolutely feel some short-term degree of happiness, especially if you were cold, naked, and hungry. Long-term, life-defining happiness will be difficult to come by on the physiological needs level. You can work up the levels and ask the same question: is the requisite components to create and maintain short and lifelong happiness present? I think you may be on to the point that I am trying to make but let's keep on it. You can see that one thing should start becoming increasing clear, that happiness is incredibly individualistic, that one person's requirements to achieve happiness may be far different than the next. Some people are happy with a stick. Other people want a limited-edition turbo-charged

Tesla with a built in prostate massager that can be controlled by an iPhone app.

Whether you are high maintenance or low, there are requirements that must be met in order to achieve lasting, long-term happiness or life satisfaction. Certainly, your physiological and safety needs must be met. It's hard to be happy and hungry or happy and scared. Once a person secures the necessities and provides safety, they reach the love and belonging section of the hierarchy, which, I believe, is the foundry of happiness. This is where we gain friendships, find love and intimacy, and develop a family. I think that many would agree that this level would add the missing puzzle piece that would allow them satisfaction, while others would feel the need to reach for more, the respect, strength, freedom, and recognition that could be found on the next level of the pyramid. There are no wrong answers, just requirements that you personality holds, which will determine your level of happiness. If you are a driven person, a real get-goer, you may not feel satisfied until you reach a high self-esteem, or position of strength, which will take longer or require more to feel the same level of happiness of someone who finds theirs in family or friends.

Now that we've broadly defined what we as human beings require in reaching a level of happiness, if we get all that stuff, we will be happy, right? The answer is no. If you to the store to prepare for Thanksgiving dinner and you buy the turkey and the dressing, the yams and potatoes, everything on the exhaustive list you printed out so you wouldn't forget anything, not even the canned jellied cranberry sauce, which is the best by the way, then you took all those bags home and plopped them on the dining room table, would you be ready to eat? The fact of the matter is, even if you meet your needs and check all of the boxes, there is still a choice that needs to be made; you have to opt in to happiness. Trying to get two scientists/researchers/psychiatrists to agree upon where exactly happiness comes from and how to tap into it is like trying to arrange a coffee klatch with Axl Rose and Slash.

This is the point of the discussion that the wheels start to get a bit wobbly, so I'll just say a bunch of words in a random order and hope that at some level they make sense. Modern science, through research, has shown that happiness has widespread impact through most of the major areas of the brain, especially the left prefrontal cortex, but has fallen short of pinpointing exactly where it originates. That's probably because there's a lot of shit up in there, nerves and receptors, capacitors and sprockets, and they all have different jobs, making understanding the creation of happiness as equally perplexing as the creation of depression. We do know that the limbic system of the brain, or as I like to call it, the paleo-mammalian cortex, deals with emotions, among about a billion other things. I feel that both depression and happiness come from the same neighborhood where they probably went to rival schools and competed for the same girl, who chose the depression, because he's the bad boy.

So, how can some people have everything, money, opportunity, visible abdominal muscles, and be miserable a-holes, while others who live frugally, within far simpler means and meager possessions display genuine happiness and contentment? The simple and clearest answer is that they choose to be happy. Now I will tell you, nothing makes me want to chop someone across the trachea more than when they say "Depression is a mood" or "Just choose happiness." As much as it fucking galls me to do, I have to admit that those organic smelly dirt eaters were right. You can just choose to be happy. Of course, it's not as easy as all that but it's not all that hard either. You simply make a mindful commitment to living and choosing happy. You appreciate and feel content with where you are, even if it's not where you want to end up eventually. Over time, choosing to be happy will lead to the belief that you are happy, which will lead to a healthy appraisal of your overall life satisfaction or long-term happiness.

Now, I have cared for my needs big and small. I have provided assets and resources, gained friends, and grown my family, and now I actively choose happiness. What about depression? I said earlier that it is possible for a person to be happy and depressed at the same time, and I believe it, however, where you have a choice in being happy, your clinical depression gives zero shits about what you want. What sick fucker wouldn't opt out of depression if given the opportunity? Maybe those masochists who hang from hooks for fun, and maybe Bill Cosby? Listen, if you're fighting for your very life and are surrounded by black sadness, smelling the flowers and taking inventory of all of your blessings will simply have to wait until the storm clears, which makes happiness seem even farther removed, even harder to get to. That being said, some of the most genuinely happy people I have ever met in my life were sufferers like you and me, and the reason is elegant in its simplicity. We appreciate the light. We appreciate happiness so profoundly because of what we had to go through to experience it.

When you suffer from depression it's not like flipping a coin, "heads," I'm going to feel happy; "tails," it's back to Bizarro Narnia, where everything sucks. We don't get a membership card to "happy" to use when we're not currently suffering. We still have to choose to be happy, just like everyone else, but sometimes we have to do it under fire. I take great joy in finding happiness throughout my day, a cup of coffee in the morning, or a kiss on the cheeks and booty squeeze in the afternoon, maybe a warm hug toward evening. I take perhaps my greatest joy in my belief that despite my pain and suffering, despite the years of dark torment, that I am a happy person, that I have found meaning and enjoyment that have transcended my negative trajectory.

So I will flash you a "peace sign" while I braid wildflowers in my long unwashed hair and simply say, "Just choose happiness, man. Just choose happiness."

Hello, my friend. How are you? It's always good to see you, I mean, talk to you in the morning. Have you ever just woken up and wondered what in the name of Queen Hippolyta of the Amazons is going on with your life? The world seems like one never-ending paradox of health-induced sickness. We walk around all day in masks to protect our health while feeling sicker and sicker on the inside, especially between our ears. It gets frustrating and challenging, even more so when you're trying to work through a mental health crisis, with PTSD, and do work and prepare for a really important therapy appointment tomorrow. Whoa, kind of let 'er run free there for a minute, sorry about that. It just seems like were playing in a high-stakes game with marked cards and a stacked deck, and if we some-how miraculously win a hand, they will shoot us in the patella, and if we're lucky, they'll hit it.

I used to have a system where I would just write the day off, be a bitchy little whiner, then move on, but I'm all about working on shit now, so let's get to work. Some days I wake up raw, just thinking about the personal mountain I need to climb before I can climb the regular life mountain that lies just beyond. I just experi-ence moments of intense frustration followed by utter hopelessness that just robs me of my strength and will. Deep breath. I'm going to change my tack slightly to try to redirect my attention. Have you ever heard about the paradox of shutdown? I would have been sur-prised if you would have said yes. It's a paradox that basically states that when a person feels depression what they want most to do in this world is to shutdown, to withdraw from society, to go live in a cave.

The paradox comes from the knowledge that in the darkness of the cave that we long for lives the beast who will feed on us, which will want to makes us withdraw further. I know that paradox sucks, but wait, there's more. There's another depression paradox called the paradox of effort, which states that to neutralize the effects of depression takes significant sustained effort, but depression drains all available energy, hence the paradox. Depression is such a goddamn pain in the fuck, sometimes.

Wasn't I just talking about being happy just like a couple of pages ago? Welcome to the wide world of dysfunction, next up, speed guilt and shame. I feel better just venting for a minute. The fact is there is nothing really wrong other than a general disgust for having to deal with depression every day of my life, which gets super old, but I'm getting back to myself. I always feel badly when my depression gets the better of me. I feel a weakness and a guilt that I know are justified to a degree, but feels is feels. Do you know, however, what I love? I love me a good segue, so I'm going to take the opportunity that losing my mind a little has presented to me and am going to talk about a very important aspect that seems to go hand in hand with depression, and that's guilt.

Let me make one thing clear from the outset. I have been dealing with guilt and its related neurosis for far longer than I have been dealing with depression, and that is a long fucking time. Things used to be so much different when I was a kid, back then with kids raised in the church using guilt was a legit parenting technique. My mom was a Jedi master at using guilt as a motivation and manipulation tool with me and my siblings. With just a few words, she could send us into an introspective journey toward redemption. I know that sounds bad, but it wasn't. She wasn't some evil puppet master pulling strings, and I have always just been very easily swayed by guilt. I have always wanted to please people and have always despised to my very core disappointing people, and when you have those traits, you are a walking "perfect storm" of potential guilt.

I don't remember the first time that I felt guilt. Does anybody? No, really, I'm curious. I do remember sitting through children's church and learning all the shit that you should feel guilty for doing, and that by doing them, you are disappointing God, and I'm like, "You had me at disappointing God." If I thought an impure thought, I felt guilty. If I didn't share, I felt guilty. I was trying to hold myself to an impossible standard, just so I didn't disappoint anyone or God. As I got older and developed, I brought my guilt along with me, as I can't remember a time in my life when I was far from it. Then the depression thing happened, and it was like the darkness just curled up inside the guilt like a giant hermit crab of malaise.

I don't believe that my depression was borne out of extreme guilt, but I feel that it found its strength and greatest ally when the two came together. This is, of course, before the crushing anxiety became depression's best friend and left guilt on the outside looking in, which guilt didn't like one little bit, so guilt did what guilt does and confronted depression, who was like, "Leave me out of this," and now it's just awkward whenever the three get together. My guilt just made it a very comfortable environment for my depression and advantageous position from where to launch offensives. Here's the deal, though, I'm not a dick; at least I try not to be. I know I'm easily subjected to guilt responses, and so I go through life trying to be the best person that I can be, knowing that the only sure way to not obsess about screwing up is to be forgiven by the person whom I disappointed. It's true. If I feel guilty about a shortcoming I had with someone, I will fixate and worry about that one single instance until they tell me that it's okay, even if it's so small, they look at me like I have a pickle growing out of my forehead when I tell them.

The combination of guilt and depression is powerful. It has killed many people over the years and is to be taken lightly at your own peril. It's not just generalized guilt. There are some specific guilt areas that seem to attach themselves individually to sufferers of depression, especially those who are in relationships and have families. When you have others who rely on you, it significantly ramps up the pressure to perform, to earn, to manage, and with that pressure comes stress, and not far behind lurk anxiety and depression. Relationship guilt happens when we don't feel like we are living up to the high standards that we set for ourselves, then when depression hits, it takes us even farther away from where we feel we should be, where we are needed. The debilitating impact of depression takes us away from our friends and family, even if we're in the same room, and it makes us feel we are constantly letting the most important people in our lives down, which makes us feel even guiltier, which feeds the monster. I think you get the point. It's a real lose-lose situation, where you mostly lose.

My torment isn't limited to the house and activities and events within. I experience an overall feeling of unpreparedness and incompletion in most facets of my life. I constantly feel like I should be doing more than I am both professionally and personally to help achieve a greater degree of security for our family. I can't tell you how many times I have told Lisa that she'd be far better off away from me or how the boys would benefit from the nondepressed influence of a strong male role model. When I said that it was something that I believed, I wasn't just saying it for argument purposes, which is so fucked up because how far gone do you have to be to tell your wife, whom you love dearly, that she should find some other cock and balls. Sometimes it gets to the point where you can't tell where one neurosis ends and the others begin. They all just meld into a dense fog of uneasy apprehensiveness and foreboding.

One of the greatest cruelties that I have ever known personally is in the feeling of guilt for having depression. I know that depression is not a choice, that it is a mental health disorder that offered me no input before it changed my life forever, but it doesn't matter if I understand it or not. It still feels natural for me to feel regretful about how my depression affects other around me. There is a feeling of unworthiness as it relates to my guilt and depression, like I don't merit any resources that would offer me help and support. I think that it is becoming increasing clear what big impact guilt can have. How it can go from a desire to not disappoint people to an accomplice in the unraveling of a person's reality.

I think that I've talked to you at some point about my aversion to certain scents, and what I'm really talking about is my aversion of having someone else smell me. Unless I smell good, then you can sniff away. I'm not a fan of body odor, which is why you won't find me at midsummer outdoor grunge festivals and chili cook-offs, but

I like to work out and I sweat a lot, which is concerning, because the thought of someone *having* to smell me bothers me greatly. I feel the same way with my depression; I don't want people *having* to deal with *my* depression. If you choose to work out with me or are working out in a gym with other people, then you're accept a certain level of nose risk, you are purposely going in harm's way, but if I then, without freshening up, go get stuck in a crowded elevator between floors, then I feel guilt for forcing my smell upon innocent people who just wanted to go down or up. Those who choose to stand by me know about my depression and expect to be exposed to some degree, but I'm crushed when my depression escapes the bounds of my containment and impacts others in any degree.

So we feel guilt for being depressed. Even though we have no choice, we feel guilt for our weakness when we let the depression affect us, and even guiltier each day that passes where we can't kick it off and move forward. We feel guilty for taking energy away from others or special times, and the list goes on and on, and I'm being serious. I can literally keep going for at least a couple more paragraphs, but I think you get the idea.

Now that I've shown the problem and what a tsunami of emotional baggage it can produce. Let's just see if we can solve it and make the world a better place. Guilt, as paraphrased from its Wikipedia page, is an emotional experience that happens when a person feels, whether it's true or not, that they have compromised their standards of conduct or moral principles and bear responsibility for that violation. Now I'm not going to say that my version of that definition would be accepted by all brain-ologists, but I think it has a ticket to the ballpark, so it'd be sitting in there somewhere. That being said, in its simplest form, guilt is formed by the compromising of personal standards. What that tells me is that I feel in some way that I have compromised my high ethical standards by contracting the social disease of depression. I know I can't do the new bullshit math, but even my old mathematical configurations have something not quite adding up in this equation.

There is a massive, gaping x that needs to be solved for in order for the formula to figure correctly and make sense of. The problem lies in the knowledge that the *x* stands for something that is unquantifiable; it stands for stigma. Now if you don't know what stigma is, I'm not talking about Beelzebub writing shit on your skin from the inside, which would be unsettling. What I'm talking about is public disapproval based on a physical or psychological characteristic. Depression had been stigmatized for generations upon generations before Ma Deever's oldest son contracted it by chewing some old gum he found next to a mud puddle. I need to tell myself again, and again, and at least once more that I *did not choose to be depressed*, or be impacted by depression, and that depression is a mental health condition not something you become infected with while on shore leave visiting pleasure island.

We have to change paradigms about how people think and what they feel about depression in our world. When it comes to this issue, we're still burning witches at the stake and lighting the fire by rubbing stones together, it's embarrassing. No person should, either consciously or unconsciously, feel compulsory guilt because they are unlucky enough to be clinically depressed. This bullshit has got to stop, and from where I sit, there is only one way to do it, and I've been trying to make that happen for quite a while. We all need to *talk*, we all need to *communicate*, and we need to begin a global conversation about how we think about and treat those who suffer with depression.

Nothing is going to be easy when it comes to depression society has cognitive dissonance, meaning that there is widespread understanding of the causation and science around the condition of depression but also the people who suffer feel guilt derived from social stigma that has been deeply ingrained within us. I will stand, I will tell my story, and I will change the way that I see and treat my depression. It is not my fault. By feeling guilt, I am perpetuating the stigma, and I will no longer be a part of the problem.

It's not about getting rid of guilt. Guilt is an emotion that comes preinstalled on most makes and models of human beings. There is guilt that has been absolutely earned, every atom bought and paid for by misdeeds and less than pure intent. This is not about living a guilt-free life; it is about knowing the difference between guilt that has been earned and deserved and guilt that has no rightful place in our lives and in our struggles, which robs us of strength and dignity.

I appreciate you sticking with me today. They aren't all wins. Sometimes everything tastes salty because you spend the day pissing into the wind. This is life on the dark side. You never quite know what each new day will bring, what kind of emotions will come into play. You just keep going and hope that some of the shit you throw against the wall will form a complete picture for someone. I know that I've been talking about guilt, a lot of guilt, but I haven't talked about a special box on a shelf somewhere deep in a storage closet in my brain where I have been collecting a special guilt for many years. This is where I keep all of my Joshua guilt separate and organized and waiting to be dealt with. I really want to deal with this box. I want to be able at some point to move beyond the hold it has over my life, and I want to feel like I've done all that I could do to make Josh's life everything that he deserves it to be.

I'm not going to open this box today. I am far too emotional. If I was forced to tell the truth I would say that most days I am far too emotional to deal with the contents that lie within. I know that there is probably a bunch of guilt in there that doesn't belong to me, some that I collected others that I appropriated. Someday I truly hope to be rid of the box, but as I think about it, I feel that this dysfunction that I have, this emotive sensitivity, is my closest connection with my son, and not having it around, no matter the emotional burden, scares me greatly, like by doing so in some way I am severing a connection, and I just can't bear it right now.

THURSDAY, JULY 23, 2020

Hey, good morning, and good news. By making it through yesterday, we won a brand-new day! That's how we do it. We live and breathe and deal with what comes up, then we take care of ourselves and meditate and do everything we can possibly do be successful. Some days we fall short, some days we fall far short, but we never stop, we never ever give up or in. I didn't struggle to get out of bed today. I didn't give myself the opportunity. I just sat up and got moving, each step toward that fresh cup of freshly brewed perkaliscious-ness. I just made that word up and now own all exclusive rights. Before I get to that fresh caffeinated capitalism, there are three of man's best fiends that have a road that needs a good smelling, so I get them all leashed up and we head out. The sun hasn't quite made a proper appearance, but the cobalt blues and magentas are giving way to softer, more pastel colors every passing minute. Even though the summer solstice was barely a month ago, you can start to feel the darkness holding on a little bit longer every morning.

Hondo peed on Maudie's head this morning, not on purpose; at least I don't think it was on purpose. He is constantly trying to keep and increase the territory within his empire, which means that if it sticks in the ground or stands still, it has to be marked, annexed, and taxed into the Holy Hondo Empire and toe-licking emporium. Maudie just happened to be giving a sniff to a mailbox post at the same time the Emperor reclaimed it as sovereign ground. Other than some run-of-the-mill cranial urination, the walk concluded without incident, and after a quick cleaning, I found myself holding my favorite mug, soft music playing in the background. Ghosts of yesterday still resonate with me, and I need to shake them off. Apparently I still suffer from hangovers. I need to move beyond my attitude and level of upset about the guilt issue. If you could only imagine the hours in my life that I have spent feeling guilty, the sheer amount of wasted effort. It's like being a government contractor but with ethical standards.

Today is my final scheduled meeting with Dr. K, not my last meeting, just the last one based on my mental setback and PTSD. It feels like a year ago when I first sat down to talk with you. I know it must feel like that to you. I am so positive about my mindfulness and the work that I have been accomplishing regarding the anxiety and PTSD. I have learned so much that I was unaware was happening just behind the curtain. It hasn't been easy at any point. I have had to redefine my whole processing process. It's funny. I just got this little twinge of missing something, you know that feeling you get sometimes on the last day of a killer vacation when you know you have to go home the next day. That's a unique experience in dealing with affairs of the brain, especially for me.

I have been in this fight for a long time, long enough to know that there is nothing that is going to offer the hope of a cure, that my depression will be there with me on the last day I roam this earth, looking for smaller dinosaurs to eat. At points over the many years, I have treated it as a prison sentence, from the context of severity and duration, not from a quality of life point of view. I wasn't eating bologna on white bread, making wine in my toilet, or keeping an eye on my sweet ass. It was often just easier to tell myself that it wasn't going to get any better, and it was going to be around forever. I know I have said this before, or maybe not. There is only so many words rattling around upstairs that I assume the same ones come out from time to time, like when you're playing Bingo and every goddamn game they call B4, then make some Bingo joke about it. Sometimes when you feel a little hope or things get better, it fills you with dread because you only want to get better if you can stay better. There is nothing more soul-crushing than hope revoked, feeling warming rays of sunshine on your cheeks after a long dark night; only to have it blotted out by another dark cloud is demoralizing and dangerous.

When I started this process weeks ago, it was with the mindset that I was going to make changes that would be lasting, or I wasn't going to do it. I will not put myself through the emotional meat grinder of experimentation any more. I want to work toward a goal of relief and pain management that was achievable and realistic. Now that I have achieved that goal to a degree, I just want to keep it going, keep moving forward actively dealing with my issues, and I really think that is one of the topics that I will be talking with Dr. K about later. In actuality, I already know the answer. I just find it reassuring to hear it from someone in a position of authority, like when an airline pilot comes on the intercom after some unexpected turbulence and reassures you that mathematically you have a great chance of not dying.

I finish my last swig of coffee and get momentum working in my favor. I still have to work out and work in, meaning get some paperwork processed and some emails responded to, before the big meeting. I'm telling you, one of my favorite feelings in the world is the "just got done with a hard workout" feeling. It makes me feel fresh and clean even though I'm sweaty and smelly and gives me energy to sit down and file paperwork and sound like I'm a professional when I compose a work email. I feel some nervous energy building as the day moves toward my Zoom with Dr. K, like there is significant weight of importance for this meeting, like if it doesn't go well, all my work to this point would be invalidated. That's what it feels like, the final oral exam of a tough class, and that it counts for like 96 percent of the overall class grade. I always hated situations like that because we all knew that one jackwagon who could do the bare minimum all semester long, then nail the exam and pull an A, and another poor soul who works hard, pours their all into the work, but bombs the test and the class.

I need to just relax because this isn't an all-or-nothing type of situation. If I had taken a significant step back, we'd just schedule another meeting. I wouldn't lose my ability to walk around in free society or have to report as registered sense offender and inform my neighbors. I long to be given a "clean bill of health," or at least a version of that. I want Dr. K to smile that wry smile and tell me, "Well, it looks like you're doing good, you're on a good path, just keep walking it." That kind of thing. I think my recent mood fluctuations have given me pause and made me think I'm not as far along as I hoped to be, but I have to understand that is going to happen, and I need to be practicing that self-compassion, continuing down the good path. Deep centering breathes, feel better, and think better.

I get my home recording studio all set up. I take my laptop down the hall to Josh's room, away from yapping dogs, and prop the door shut. I adjust the lighting, so I look less like someone testifying against the mob and more like someone talking to his doctor, through a computer, which really will be more of a thing going forward than anyone realizes at this point. Five minutes early is right on time. I know that she won't be giving away time for free, so I have five minutes to spend in the waiting room. I check myself, just in case I was about to wreck myself. Hair look on, no visible nose hairs, no remnants of lunch lingering on the front grill, my shirt is properly buttoned, and my collar is passable. For some reason, don't ask me why, but I can't stand when the collar of my shirts is limp or wrinkled; it just messes with my head. The shirt itself can be wrinkled—hell, it can have bloodstains and a sleeve ripped off from a rogue badger attack, and I don't care—but if the collar is all floppy, then it will irritate me to no end. No such worries today, and since this is the last time I will be "seen" in any official capacity today, the shirts coming right off at the conclusion of this meeting anyway.

At the top of the hour, almost to the second, there are suddenly two participants in the meeting, and the clock has started. Dr. K looks both businesslike and relaxed, projecting a feeling of both comfort and professional authority. Like with every session, we begin with the exchange of pleasantries and a recap of what was talked about at our last session, before moving to a rundown of what has transpired over the last two weeks. As much as I want to get that pat on the head while she says "Good boy," it can't come at the expense of the truth, or because I glossed over the difficulty that I've had. If nothing else, I would rather border on exaggeration in describing my challenges with the idea that it may spur us to try something else or not. So I tell her how I have experienced some recent frustrations, and then I describe my feelings to her. As much as I like her and appreciate her knowledge and insights, it's a minor annoyance when I talk, and she nods and takes notes without verbally responding. I don't know if I should just keep talking, even though my train of thought has pulled into the station and let everyone off, or if I should sit quietly and wait for her to comment. I opt for the latter and just sat their quietly, like an awkward trained walrus waiting to be tossed a fish.

She breaks the silence after what seem like minutes but in actuality were like ten seconds, and I can tell that she has a bunch of stuff to say and is in the process of getting in put in order. She begins by asking me about my depression triggers, assuming that I've been around the block enough times that she doesn't have to ask me if I know what a depression trigger is, even though it is pretty self-explanatory. The deal with depression triggers, in my mind, is that they are like the inside of a shark's mouth. You have the big mambo's up front. Those are the big issues that will tip the scales toward depression no matter how stable a person may have been feeling. Those big things include grief and loss, life transition, illness, money problems, and addiction, to name a few. These big issues are usually pretty obvious and, in my opinion, not the most dangerous of triggers. If a person has an established support structure around them, the big issues get a spotlight and get talked about and dealt with.

The secondary triggers, the second and third rows of flesh shredding shark teeth are the real killers because often these triggers go unnoticed or played down until they break the proverbial dromedary vertebrae. These secondary triggers may include some general to all like stress, lack of sleep, change in diet, rejection of some kind, and more individual and unique ones like, conflict with a coworker or neighbor, a losing effort by a favorite team, or even a change in technology or internet access. Sometimes, however, there isn't one singular "trigger." Sometimes it is an accumulation of frustrations that all of a sudden boils vigorously, creating a "plethora of triggers." It's not a gaping wound that easily explainable and understandable. It's death by a thousand cuts, where you didn't see them or feel them until after you were already bleeding. Sometimes life itself and all the countless bullshit intricacies that seem to pile up around our feet are the biggest and most unavoidable triggers of them all.

I work through my thought progression with Dr. K, and she nods and makes notes on her pad. We don't spend too much time dwelling on my "triggers." I think that I've demonstrated to her that I am not only keenly aware of my triggers, that I, at least of late, have been proactive in managing my exposure to them, which I feel is unquestionably true. You don't go into any fight without knowing your weaknesses just as thoroughly as you understand your strengths. Do you think that Captain Kirk just had to take off his shirt to defeat the Gorn? No, he had to rely on his wits and knowledge of seventeenth-century gunsmithing and black-powder-manufacturing practices, which others at Starfleet Command may have seen as a shortcoming.

She asks if I have ever heard of double depression, and I give her a quizzical look, like when a dog thinks they hear the word "treat" or "walk." To me it sounds like the worst sitcom ever on the Lifetime Network starring Joaquin Phoenix and Winona Ryder about a couple living in a minivan by a river. I was way off. Double depression is what Dr. K thinks that I actually suffer from, and it's a combination of two types of depression. The first is a type called persistent depressive disorder (PDD) which is characterized as less severe but chronic depression that has lasted over two years. I'm not "down with PDD," especially the less severe part, but I got the chronic thing covered, but as the late-night pitchmen say, and Dr. K would echo, "But wait there's more." There's this other kind of depression called major depressive disorder (MDD), which I am totally aware of as it is in my file in multiple places. MDD is exactly what you would expect, significantly impactful depressive episodes that can be utterly debilitating to the person experiencing it. Double depression would be a combination of the two types, chronic manageable depression with occurrences of severe major depression, and everything about it rings true to my situation. Of course, the only real thing that would change would be a heading in my file. It wouldn't change my course of treatment options or give me a tax write-off; it just increases my understanding of what I personally deal with. "Oh, you just suffer from depression, that's cute, me? Well, I don't want to make a big deal about it or anything, but I have double depression. I know. If you want, I can autograph your Prozac bottle."

I know that she has more to say on the topic of my frustrations, but I get the feeling that she would like to save that until the big wrap up, so she asks me about my mom and if I'd spent any time down by the river. I tell her I haven't but not because closure isn't important to the human condition, it certainly is, but like my big box of Josh guilt, I keep my mom close by purposely not going to the river. I know that this is not ideal from the psychological point of view, and I need to fulfill a promise made. I just don't know if emotionally I can bear it at this particular point in time. Dr. K understands and mentions that she doesn't feel that it is crucially important to my situation right now. This is something that will happen in due course and will be profound when it does, but because of its significance, it shouldn't be rushed or forced into completion.

We talk about how my mindfulness is going, if I'm still spend-ing time in meditation and contemplation, and I tell her that I am. In actual fact, I have become an absolute believer in mindfulness and the impact that it can have when it comes to anxiety. I think there is nothing healthier that a person can do for their overall mental state than to explore their thoughts and feelings on a regular basis, and keep in mind that this is coming from someone who, prior to a few weeks ago, was so removed from his own thoughts and feelings, he could be legally be declared void. This makes Dr. K smile, hear-ing that I have continued my healthy practice, even in the face of adversity has told her something that she needed to hear, and maybe I did too. I know I have been guilty in the past of continuing a healthy practice until I hit the first roadblock, then dropping it like it was made of gluten. I actually can't see myself not meditating at any point. It makes me feel that good.

I glance at my watch and I know that our time is running short, and I think Dr. K senses that shift in the dynamic. She starts to leaf through her notebook, trying to find that thing that she wanted to revisit from earlier. She tells me that I shouldn't be overly concerned with getting frustrated from time to time. It happens to even the strongest of humans. The trick is to keep doing things that move you forward emotionally and psychologically, to continue on the path of health both physically and mentally. She tells me that in her opinion that I don't require any more than routine maintenance therapy sessions unless something unforeseen arose or my situation changed. Then she tells me something that hit me between the eyes. She says, "With depression there is no finish line. It's what makes it so evil, by persevering you have given yourself the chance to work through hard times and difficulties, which has made you stronger than you know. Just keep going."

I got my pat on the head and much more. I say a very heartfelt goodbye and promise to make another appointment in a month or two, and with a click, I am out of the meeting and standing alone in Big J's room. Unlike the meetings before, I don't need to process any information or work out any ancillary feelings. I feel that I had reached an emotional terminus, so I close the laptop and make my way down the hall. I plug the computer into its "docking station," which is basically just the four dollar plastic Walmart storage bin that I use as my elevated desk, sitting next to an outlet. I find Lisa folding clothes in the laundry room and tell her about the meeting. I know that convincing her that lasting change is happening will take some time and effort. She has been with me for far too long to walk out on that limb, no matter how much she wants it to be true.

It's been a long day. You don't realize how physically tiring emotionality can be. I decide to end the day with a cup of coffee. I know its pushing zero hour, and I may pay a price for my folly as I lay my head on the pillow, but it seems like the right thing to do, and as it turns out, I'm a "good boys," so I celebrate.

FRIDAY, JULY 24, 2020

Good to see you this fine day. Today is going to be a little bit different than the others so bear with me, but I promised myself something and today's payday. You see, back after my first therapy session weeks ago, I had some inner dialogue about seeing the process through, working hard and giving it all I had to give. I really didn't need extra motivation as I was fully committed to the process from day one, but a little bonus never killed anyone, right? Wrong, apparently a bonus did kill someone, and a veteran to boot. Back in World War I, there was these things called adjusted compensation certificates, or "bonuses," issued to veterans during the Great Depression that weren't redeemable until 1945, but veterans marched on Washington, DC, in 1932 demanding immediate bonus payments because of extreme financial hardship. They camped out in shanties next to the capital and protested daily. When the US House of Representatives voted to reject the immediate payment, many of the protesters revolted. Herbert Hoover and Douglas MacArthur drove out the interlopers using tear gas and tanks to destroy their makeshift abodes. One of the protesters was shot to death, because of a bonus, which now kinda casts a pall over where I was going, or maybe a moment of silence will help.

Where was I going with the bonus anyway? Thanks for bringing me back. I told myself If I made it through the process that I could reward myself by bitching about whatever I wanted to, that I could just open up the vault and air out my smelly drawers, that were filled with things that irritate me. So that's what I'm going to do. I'm going to have an old-fashioned whine-o-rama before getting back to the regular programming.

Cold coffee pisses me off. There is never a reason to drink cold coffee. If circumstances merit you leaving your coffee until it goes cold, like you're arm just fell off, or the Jehovah's Witnesses were having a pledge drive or some shit and wouldn't leave until you drew a sidewalk chalk pentagram on your porch, lit some candles, and grabbed Woodrow, your pet chicken, then make some fresh coffee. If nothing else, throw it in the nuker and hit a button. Keep in mind that if you settle for cold coffee, then you'll settle for anything, and before you know it, Girl Scouts will be riding roughshod over you and you'll have "tagalongs" and "samoas" coming out your ass until next spring. Conversely, if you are drinking "cold brew" coffee, you should guard against it getting warm at all costs, and never, ever just leave your coffee unattended in a car; it's just irresponsible.

I hate standing in lines. I know that modern life requires you to stand in a line from time to time, whether it's to check in for a flight or hotel or check out after buying cheese doodles. We all stand in lines, but for the love of buttered monkeys, please stop doing these things, people. Stop complaining about standing in line or about the speed in which it's moving. We are all aware of the situation and don't need constant reminders every thirty seconds. Be a responsible queue-stander and know what you want when you get to the front and be ready to order and pay expeditiously. Don't be one of those oblivious assholes who get to the front then wonder what they want. Don't cut or ask to cut. Your time isn't any more valuable than the rest of ours Rockefeller. Lastly, if you have to be on the phone while in line, don't act like you're the only person who knows someone not in the line and flaunt your "popularity" by carrying on a loud one-way conversation for all to hear. Nobody cares.

I hate three-way light switches. I know I got your attention ever so briefly there, but three-way switches are such a pain in the ass. You flip a switch, and nothing happens, so you have to walk down the hall and flip the switch, then go back to the original switch and flip it back to the original position and pray to God Almighty that nobody hits the other switch resetting the whole process. Like I said earlier, my house was wired by Clark W. Griswold, so every time you flip a switch it's an adventure.

I hate selfies, and yes, I hate myself for taking them. Selfies aren't going away anytime soon, and I see myself taking more as photogenic situations present themselves, like if I'm in Yellowstone and I see one of the animatronic buffalos they have programmed to wander the park, I'm going to want to get as close as humanly possible for that photo op, maybe even climb on its back and ride it like Mongo from Blazing Saddles, even though I know he rode a longhorn steer. If you're going to take a selfie, don't make stupid faces or micromanage the situation, treat taking a selfie like farting. You want to limit people's exposure to it at all costs, unless you're a selfish prick.

I hate long phone calls. If I can't communicate what I need to in ten minutes or less, then I feel that I need to adjust my mode of communication. Now I need to justify this statement to a degree. If I'm conducting a meeting with a client over the phone because we couldn't get together in person or in Zoom, then a longer call is in order, but outside that, know that my first objective when making or answering a call is working out how to get off that call at my first opportunity. Also, please also stop telling me that my "call is important" when I'm on hold. I think we both know that isn't the case, or you wouldn't keep trying to push me to the website for answers and at least have the common fucking courtesy to have more than one song or piece of music for hold cues, making people listen to the same goddamn thing for forty minutes sounds like a solid defense strategy against a manslaughter charge.

I hate group texts and emails. Now I know that group communications serve a purpose from time to time, but even so, don't just throw someone in a group without talking to them first, because there is a chance that they hate group texts and emails. Someone will ask a question, then you spend the next two hours checking dings on your phone because everyone feels like they need to respond or comment, and then you start losing chronological order, and you have to rewind the thread to see where the hell this or that is coming from and who was talking about using a corn dog as a handle for cotton candy, and there is always that one person who doesn't quite get that we all aren't insomniacs with nothing better to do than check our phones at all hours of the day and night.

I hate when people don't acknowledge kind gestures. You hold the door open for them, and they walk in without even a nod of appreciation? Oh shit, you must be Burt Reynolds or Rosie O'Donnell or someone equally important that my tingling nether regions should be thanks enough for my simple act of humanity. Listen, if you're waiting to pull into traffic and I leave you room, I'm not doing that because of who you are; I'm doing it because we're all in this together, and we should be kind to one another, and that includes not being a self-important butt-hole.

I hate spiders. I know they're beneficial, but so are vegetables.

I hate vegetables.

I hate when men are oversensitive on social media. I'm not an old-school macho, grunting, toolbelt-wearing Cro-Magnon. I believe that men should absolutely have a sensitive side, but that side should be treated like the power to summon the ghost of Jim Varney, used sparingly, if at all. The first couple of times, it will seem novel or touching, then it just gets pathetic, and before you know it, you're either crying because the horsies on the Budweiser commercial are so magnificent or are saying "Know what I mean, Vern?" after every statement you make. Either way, you are irritating those around you and embarrassing your family.

I hate having to poop in public restrooms. The only thing worse is feeling the urge and not having a bathroom around, but that another topic for another day. The problem is that most establishments try to minimize the square footage of "nonpaying" areas like bathrooms, but maximize the number of plumbing fixtures they can fit within them. So the stalls are packed tight, making it difficult to keep all your stuff on your side. Sometimes there are large gaps where the doors and stall walls meet, totally invalidating the need for the door altogether, because there's really nothing quite as awkward as making eye contact with someone who's currently dropping kids at the pool. If I'm in a stall, and there are several vacant, *do not* sit next to me, always leave a buffer when possible, and remember, unless you are a total psychopath asshole, the only acceptable communication *ever* allowed is if you made the rookie mistake of not checking TP levels when you sat down, and find yourself paperless, then you can ask your neighbor, but all other communication is forbidden.

I hate fitted sheets. Once it's on, I have no problem, but getting to that point can be a scene from *The Three Stooges*. Doing it by yourself could be considered cardiovascular endurance training, doing it with your spouse could be considered couples immersion therapy. Also, there is no way to fold that goddamn thing, so it looks like you didn't just wad it up and throw it in your closet.

I hate pouring a bowl of cereal and then realizing that there is no milk in the house. There is no way to make this situation better, you can't pray about it, Go Fund Me accounts are pointless, and first responders turn a blind eye even though they are here to serve. All you can do is try to pour the cereal back in the box, which is difficult—who am I kidding, it's freaking impossible. I hear you now, just go to the Easy Mart and get some milk. What world do you live in where that ever works out? Everyone knows that by the time you get back the cereal compulsion will have subsided and all that will be left in its place is unrequited angsty inconclusiveness.

I hate painting. I really enjoy from time to time sitting down with a fresh canvas and palette and letting creativity happen, but if you want me to choose a color and paint a wall, that shit just isn't gonna happen. There have been zero rooms I have entered in my life where I've thought to myself, "I would love to paint this room," and I've been to LAX. First off, there are too many colors, just looking at the paint chips at the hardware store makes me want to move to a cave, and prepping with tape and paper? I'll cut a bitch.

I hate getting comfortable, then needing to pee, or like I call it "an average night."

I hate socks. Socks are overrated pains in the asses. They get all loose and sloppy on your foot, squirming down hoping to get past your ankle before rounding the corner of your heel and ending up rolled up around your toes. I know that our laundry must be like turn-of-the-century tombstone because socks go missing and the ones that don't have unexplained holes in them. Again, I know that socks serve a purpose, but you either get crap or have to spend so much for a quality pair that you have to ask yourself how much you just spent on a pair of socks, like you spent how much on a pair of socks? Are you insane? Did the Publishers Cleaning House van drop by with a big check and balloons so you thought you'd celebrate by buying a pair of socks?

I hate slow drivers. Listen, I'm in this vehicle to get from point A to point B. I'm not here to experience the "joy of driving" or impress anybody with a display of responsible car handling ability. That being said, I do not drive recklessly, just impatiently. I hate tailgaters just as much as the next guy, so if you're wondering, that isn't me riding your ass. I'll just be the guy a respectful distance behind you saying, "It's the pedal on the right, Mabel." In case you were waiting for me to start complaining about people's general parking abilities or about parking lots, I actually don't hate those. For some reason, parking lots make sense to me, probably because you encounter the worst the human experience has to offer in a parking lot, it's like Thunderdome, with slightly less chainsaw.

This has been a cool little change of pace for me. Generally, I try to overlook the negative, giving preference to positive thoughts, feelings, and actions, but letting yourself vent can have positive effects if done correctly. An emotional release can lead to a catharsis or cathartic moment that has the ability liberate a person from anxiety or stress or simply make them feel better. "I'm glad I got that off my chest" is a cathartic response. Ranting can also be healthy and lead to reduced stress and a better relationship with the "listener" if done respectfully and correctly. It can also lead to far deeper shit if done incorrectly. I've found I'm equally adept at both ways, but I sleep better if I do it correctly. There is no doubt in my mind that living an encouraging, optimistic life is where I want to be. It pays far more dividends and makes me feel like an overall better person, so I'm not looking to change that. However, there are just a few more thing I would like to get off my chest, you know, just for giggles.

I hate giggling; laugh or laugh not, there is no giggle.

I hate when people don't replace the toilet paper in the bathroom, and you have to walk down the hall with your pants around your ankles to get more.

I hate cellophane tape that you can't get started.

I hate when I cut my finger- or toenails too close or when others don't throw away theirs.

I hate when you can't sharpen a pencil, the tip breaks off or it sharpens lopsided.

I hate Bluetooth phone attachment that allows you to not hold the phone while talking on it. How much does a phone weigh, you jag off? Is it worth confusing everyone around you just so you don't have to hold a phone?

I hate toothpaste rolls and when the toothpaste falls off the brush right onto your freshly ironed work shirt.

I hate cold butter; try spreading that shit on anything but wood.

I hate getting clothes stuck in zippers and weak pant crotches that prevent roundhouse kicks.

I hate depression, I hate feeling depressed, I hate being tired to the bone getting out of bed, and I hate that I have to fight every day. Nevertheless, the thing I hate most in this world, with every fiber of my being, is when depression wins, when it takes good people. It will get no satisfaction from me. All it will get is a fucking fight, and I love that.

Saturday July 25, 2020

Hello and good morning to you. Our time is drawing to a close, my friend, I'm going to spend time with you today and tomorrow, then I'm going to let you go. You have done some great work for me that I will not soon forget, and at the end of the day, there is nothing better that we can do for our fellow man than to hold out a helping hand and let them know that they are not alone. I know that holding that hand out can be scary too. Sometimes people who are drowning out of sheer panic will pull others down to the depths with them, and that needs to be guarded against, but we all need to be willing to stand in the breech with the people we love. I'll spare you the rest of my emotional discourse, at least until tomorrow. As for now, I'm thinking about coffee but looking deeply into Hondo's longing eyes, so I think I'll start the magic coffee machine and take the three impure-blooded Franken-wieners on a stroll through the moors.

I don't usually take the dogs on Saturday. The Dog Walkers Local Union 819 allows me some degree of flexibility, but it's a stunning summer morning and I'm feeling up to it, so let's earn that steaming cuppa. As we round the corner where my daily anxiety once began, I get a nostalgic twinge. It feels like it's been so long since I've dealt with some of those issues, and I've come such a long way. Now I just have the regular stress of walking three crazy small furballs through an obstacle course of unimpressed cats, industrious nut-hoarding squirrels, and un-peed-upon posts. We make it home without serious injury or leaving a dog behind, which would be bad, but I've emotionally prepared myself for such a contingency, just in case. The coffee tastes like liquid victory over a challenging foe, and enjoying it on the back patio with non-crows chirping peacefully and a sweet breeze gently lifting the wispy clouds across the horizon adds to an overall contentment that does not go unnoticed.

I still have a busy morning ahead of me. I have to try and keep up with Lisa for a workout, which gets harder and harder as there seems to be no limit for how "fit" a person can become. After that, I need to head to the grocery store for our weekly supply stock-up before the big, bad Josh comes over for his weekly visit. I have been doing more and more mindfulness training, especially around things and times where I have set traps for myself in the past, so make no mistake that at some point prior to Lisa and J pulling in, I will have centered myself. Although I haven't experienced an episode of PTSD lately, I treat it like it can happen at any moment and that it will be with me indefinitely like my depression, making what control I can achieve paramount.

We've talked about so much you and me, but as our time is coming to a close, and I would like to talk to you about something that I feel strongly about, the importance of being yourself. Now I know you've heard the famous quote by Oscar Wilde: "Be yourself, everyone else is already taken." It's cute and witty, but it is frustratingly far from reality for so many people. This is a far bigger issue than I feel people really understand or want to understand, and for those of us who deal with depression on a regular basis, being yourself is completely and utterly out of the question, but that has got to change.

Like many other elements of my life, I learned about being someone else in church before my depression skewed my view of the world. Sometimes I feel like I'm beating up on the church, like I'm bitching about promises unfulfilled or that something really bad happened within its walls, and that is not the case. The church I went to was filled with caring people trying to be the best people they could. There was just no idea of how lasting some of the untaught lessons learned stuck with an emotional child just wanting to please important people. My first "mask" I wore, I fashioned while attending children's church. That's what we do when we feel like who we are isn't quite where we feel others would like us to be. We fashion a mask with the hopes it will better represent who we think we want to be.

My parents loved the idea of their children growing up to be steadfast people of God, and I wanted so much to be able to give them that. Unfortunately, I wasn't born that way. I had far too many questions and pieces didn't seem to fit together for me. I really tried hard, but my mind simply could not focus on the spiritual. Instead I fixated on simpler things like what would happen if Marvel's Iron Fist ever fought Atlas comics hero Ironjaw? I mean, something would have to give, right? It'd be like they were having this epic battle, then time would slow down briefly as the camera would zoom in closer as Iron Fist's, um, fist approached Ironjaw's jaw. At the moment of impact, a shockwave would be created that would emanate from the point of impact outward, shattering glass and blowing shit every-where, flipping a hot dog cart over, sending wieners flying akimbo. Who won? I don't know, and it's killing me with speculation, just like all those years ago.

The truth is that religion never felt "real" to me, but I just kept trying to force it, and when that didn't work, I fashioned a mask of faux piety and would put it on Sunday mornings from nine till noon, and again on Wednesdays if there was church stuff and, of course, vacation Bible schools. I kept this mask for years and years, even as an adult, still trying to please people, still trying to fit myself into that mold. To this day, I rarely step foot inside a church, not because I don't believe. I do believe in God, but I also believe that he made me different, and that difference is not widely accepted by most "people of God." I have and inappropriate sense of humor that pairs com-plimentary with inappropriate use of the words "fuck," "shit," and "masticate," and I fucking will never wear that shitty mask ever again. It's hard to masticate.

Since I was already accustomed, to a degree, in the art of mask wearing when I experienced depression, it was a fairly natural pro-gression to incorporate the wearing of a mask during times of dark-ness or high anxiety. Let me say that I think fashioning a "mask" or "putting on a brave face" is a completely natural reaction when you don't know what else to do, when you want to be liked, when you need to fit in. Most people, especially at a young age, aren't secure enough in who they are to not have a mask that they put on at work or at school. I think that there is a point that I need to make at this, um, point, and that is that sometimes, no matter how secure you are, no matter how strong, you still need to wear a mask from time to time. If I'm in trench warfare but have promised to be at a special event, I will don a mask and fulfill my commitment rather than bail and use my depression as an excuse.

Here's the deal, people who suffer with depression have no choice but to wear a mask from time to time; there is no way around it. Life happens at the same time depression attacks. That's one of its despicable tricks, and we can withdraw and miss out, or cancel for the umpteenth time, and feel horrible, or we can grab our smile mask and head for the door. In my opinion, for what it's worth, I find it healthier to "put on the mask of false bravado" than to stay home and feel worthless; it feels more like fighting back. The whole trick is to be as authentic a person as possible, to be true to yourself and open and transparent with others, but to understand that there will be times when depression will force you to make a choice, withdraw, go forward, and show your depression to those who won't understand or appreciate it's gravity or put on a brave face and get through.

The problem for most of us depressives is that we wear a mask more and more until it becomes a challenge to keep up storylines and illusions that aren't faithful to who we really are. That is why it is so important to keep fighting for your identity. You can never lose that because when it's gone, so is what makes you unique. You have to make a clear distinction as well between image and your mask. Your mask is a Band-Aid. It's not your skin. It covers an open wound and allows you to function over a short period while permitting the underlying injury to heal. Image is a long-term façade that you build around yourself to portray that you possess an attribute that you do not have or live a lifestyle that you cannot afford. Maintaining either a mask or an image gets more difficult with every story told, and sooner or later, it becomes impossible. So just be yourself, and here are some great reasons why, in case you need more of a reasons than just me telling you.

I think the single biggest reason to be authentic with yourself is that you'll be happier. I get it, someone talks about happiness, and all you want to do is roll your eyes and throw up in your mouth a little, but there is an absolute link between believing in who you are and greater life satisfaction. I read about this study done at Tel Aviv University, in Israel, not Tel Aviv, Idaho. Regardless, what the researchers did was divide a group of participants in half, and then they put the legs in one room and the torsos in another. Just kidding, that would be gross. Half of the participants would write about a situation where they behaved authentically, meaning in accordance with their individual thoughts, values, and beliefs, while the other half would write about a time that they behaved inauthentically. As soon as they were done writing, they were given a "test" that was designed to determine their current "happiness levels," and you can probably imagine that the authentic writers scored far higher than their counterparts. I don't remember how much higher or any real specifics, but you know, look it up, if you want to.

I don't think that the link between happiness and being true to yourself can be argued or downplayed, but there are other advantages that tie in as well, like you will stop feeling like you are a fraud or a fake. Believe me when I say that I know that nobody purposefully puts on masked emotions to defraud someone, we're not running a Ponzi scheme or claiming to be Nigerian royalty in a temporary pinch. Still, when you are not truly genuine, you feel it deep inside; it's like a sliver that can't be pulled out. Along the same lines, you will find that by being honest, you will have nothing to prove. People can detect bullshit; it's a developed sense from long ago, stored in our reptilian brain. If you claim something that can't be proven or backed up, people know, and at some point, you will have to put up or shut up, and nobody really wants to walk around with that stress. We all want to lead lives of integrity, not worried that there are things that can be held against us, and one of the surest ways to guarantee that is be as you as you can possible be. If you are living proof of who you are, what can be held against you?

One byproduct of being truer to yourself is that those that align themselves with you will be your friend because of who you are, not who you are trying to depict. The only thing worse than being fake is the fake friends and relationships that go hand in hand with the image. There is something incredibly liberating in the knowledge that someone chooses to share space without preconceived appearances. I would rather have one person who knows me and believes in who I am and wants to be in my corner than a hundred who are only there because I did or said something that wasn't authentic to me. There is also something very satisfying about being trusted. It feels good, and it's true to yourself and your original programming. Trust is the absolute basis, the foundation blocks of building any relationship, and nothing breeds trust in others quite as effectively as honesty. Living your life in truthfulness no matter what that looks like will draw people who are tired with image or fakery. Think about this. What characteristic drew you most to your best friends, past or present? I'm guessing honesty or "realness" is high on that list. People don't want to feel like they're being scammed or played.

Listen, you, like me, are here for a reason, a purpose. You may not know what that purpose is at this moment, and there's nothing wrong with that; you will know it when it happens, I promise you that. I feel that no matter what a higher purpose may be, we are all here to inspire others to lead genuinely authentic lives no matter what struggles that they encounter here on earth. To be in that position, to be an influencer, you have to be confidently true to yourself. You can't lack self-confidence or confuse it for a really good story that needs form and substance to be believable. I know it sounds like you have to be some great person that has been to space or punched a communist in the vodka chute, but an authentically living you is absolutely enough to inspire someone else to be authentically them.

Depression makes it hard to be yourself. Depression makes a lot of shit hard. Keeping a mask on longer than you absolutely have to makes it harder. I know a lot of what your feeling. I get that sometimes it feels like you don't even know yourself anymore, that you've lived one lie too many. I've been there, I've done that. Be assured that who you are, who you were born, the essence of what makes you uniquely you is there, hidden perhaps under your pain and darkness, but there nonetheless. You have everything you need to find your way back, but everything begins with communication, big surprise. Communication allows you to drop you mask, to begin the process of building trust through honesty. I'm not going to lie, telling people that you haven't been fully honest is not the most pleasant of conversations, but it is essential and, if done right, will create advocates who will stand with you in your corner.

As much as we would like to be able to rewrite our stories, that isn't possible; however, what we can do is overcome our challenges and use that experience to inspire others to do the same. Look around, the world is full of assholes trying to conform to some standard preset by other assholes and mainstream and social media. There are far fewer individuals, far fewer independently thinking, uniquely goofball, badass broken, but stronger than you can imagine, real people. Start wearing your skin with pride. You've earned every inch of it. If people knew what you've gone through, the struggles you've had, and how you won't give up, then you'd be the standard that people try to achieve and rightfully so. Fucking. Own. It.

Sunday, July 26, 2020

Okay, this is it, this is our last day together, and I'm going to try to not get emotional as we spend time together. I will say that this experience has been one of the best things that has happened in my life in recent memory. I'm not going to say it's been more impactful than when my kids were born, because those were gross, stressful days filled with fluids and yelling. I don't know why everyone says, "No day was better than when my children were born." Fuck that. I've had tons of better days including that day I spent driving a screaming family home from Las Vegas, because a family road trip to Sin City seemed like a great idea. Regardless, you have helped me reset my paradigms regarding my mental health, thus changing my life forever going forward. I really hope that I can pay what you've done for me forward that I can encourage just one person to take a more proactive approach to managing their depression and take control over its debilitating effects.

I truly feel that I am a blessed man. A little over twenty years ago, I came within a breath of ending my life. Ever since then, I have done all I can to make the most of my second chance, or third, perhaps fourth chance, but If I am a lesson in anything, it's that there is never a time that you can let your guard down. Depression does not take days off, and PTSD is real, horrible thing. It's still crazy to me that this my last day, but I truly feel like it's time to move on with my life and that I'm ready to let you get back to yours. It's Sunday morning and all that I need to do to make the morning complete is to start the coffee and figure out what adventure the day holds in store for us.

Sometimes I think my coffee machine just flat out messes with me. It's like that one checker at the grocery store who knows their shift lasts for eight hours no matter how fast they work, so they don't work fast. Then, it seems, their pace actually gets slower as you get closer to the point where you start to take it a little personally. We had a real fancy coffee maker that had buttons and noises and little wand that would froth stuff up, but it died before it reached its first birthday, which was sad. Feeling a bit ripped off we opted for the basic, no-frills Mr. Coffee that has only one button, and works fine, but slow, like it has something against me. The biggest problem I have with this model is that it doesn't have the "steal a cup" feature that impatient coffee drinkers like me covet so much, so if I try and go early, it makes a huge mess, then Lisa comes out and we're back to fluids and yelling.

My patience was paid in full as the coffee was amazing and full-bodied and hot and made me tingle in excitement. I sat out this morning with a few crows and their incessant ca-caws but made the most of it, pretending that they are rare black flamingos performing their intricate mating ritual of irritating the shit out of their prospective mates. It is ridiculously hard, I'm finding, to keep my mind from wandering back to what today signifies, and I find myself getting more and more emotional, so I'm going to talk about this last topic, then together we'll close the book and move forward. I want to talk about something that is near and dear to my heart and that has most likely saved my life on more than one occasion—having a sense of humor.

Have you ever heard the idiom "laughter is the best medicine"? I have always wondered where it came from because I can't imagine a doctor or pharmaceutical company promoting something that doesn't require a copay or nonsocialized Western medicine in general. Apparently, it goes way back to the Old Testament. Proverbs 17:22 says "a merry heart doeth good like a medicine," whicheth is oldeth as fucketh. There is also evidence of King Solomon back in 931 BC having ancient Greek physicians prescribe patient suffering from ban humors visits to the Hall of Comedians, and you know Greeks kill at comedy, and tragedy. Now I'm not in a position professionally to comment on the validity of "laughter is the best medicine," but for me I can honestly say that "laughter, if nothing else, is the best coping mechanism for the harshness of depression." I know, as far as idioms go, that one sucks. Laughter has been clinically proven by people who work in clinics to reduce blood pressure, increase a person's tolerance to pain, and boost immune system performance. There was also a study done by *Playboy* or someone that showed laughing can actually make you more desirable.

Having the choice to laugh or cry, I have always chosen to laugh. What we are talking about whether you laugh or cry is a coping mechanism, but what in the name of the Great Cornholio is a coping mechanism anyway? Well, let me tell you. A coping mechanism is an individualized psychological method that we develop to fight the stresses we encounter in our daily lives. In essence it is whatever tool that we find works for us in dealing with specific stressors. Laughter and crying can be coping mechanisms as can be a lot of things like praying, problem-solving, exercising, asking for help, and taking responsibility. Honestly, there are as many ways to cope as there are problems requiring the coping, and there are good ways and bad ways, healthy mechanisms and disastrous cries for help. One thing to keep in mind that if you don't mindfully develop a coping strategy, one will be provided for you at some point; it's just better if you have some say in its development.

I never knew what a coping mechanism was back in my early depressive years. I cried a lot and realized that was not the best use of my time. Crying makes you feel sad, it keeps the darkness draped around you like a heavy velvet robe, and its impacts are not easily hidden from others, which was an absolute requirement. I learned early on that art worked a treat and was a healthy, productive coping mechanism but not very portable. I couldn't just pull an easel out of my pants in fourth-period geography and start painting. I could, however, doodle, which I did to distraction at times. Sometimes my notes weren't notes at all, just a series of scribbles and random characters with unfinished stories fighting heroically against the forces of the growing blob of ink. Humor, however, has been with me for as long as I can remember far before I knew that it could be used as a coping mechanism.

The problem with relying on humor to get through a tough day is that there is more than one kind of humor my young padawan, like with many things there is a light side and a dark side, and wielded unwisely can lead to greater difficulties. What am I talking about? Well, let me try and offer a degree of explanation. There have been a bunch of studies done on the role humor plays on every facet of the human experience, including depression. In order to fully understand its scope, you need to quantify to some degree the types of humor that exist or create some kind of humor spectrum. Researchers do this by using a scale called the Humor Styles Questionnaire developed to assess how humor is used in a person's daily life. Depending on how a person answers the questions, they are categorized into one or more of the four humor styles.

There are two positive humor types and two negative humor types, so the force is balanced, as forces should be. The two positive styles are affiliative humor, which is the tendency to share humor with others to create ease and facilitate relationships, and self-enhancing humor, which allows a person to maintain a humorous attitude even when alone and to use it as a coping tool to cheer oneself up when stressed. The dark side of comedy is comprised of aggressive humor, which is disparaging in nature used to put down or ridicule, often using offensive and racist jokes, and self-defeating humor, which tends to amuse others at a person's own expense, often to cover up true feelings at being teased or ridiculed.

Armed with this information, researches can run a variety of experiments to determine how a sense of humor impacts the human condition, but I want to talk about this one I read about in Australia that I have no source information for, but I discovered it, so. What I found amazing is that this study recruited eleven hundred fifty-four twins from Australia; that's a metric shit-ton of twins. What the researchers wanted to do was find out if people diagnosed with depression, which out of the eleven hundred, there were one hundred and forty-five with a clinical diagnosis for depression, scored higher on the two "dark" humor styles and lower on the "light," meaning was there a genetic correlation between a person's depression and the style of humor that they prefer to use.

One of the results that this study found that was unrelated to the overall purpose, but backed up the results of other studies, finding that women were two and a half times more likely to suffer from depression than men. I find that fascinating because personally I know far more men sufferers than women, which tells me that if women are indeed suffering at a higher rate, they aren't talking about it. I can hear it now. Women everywhere are saying, "Oh, we talk about it. Men just don't listen," which is true and a topic for another time.

What the study did find is that depressed people do use "self-defeating humor" more than nondepressed people and that the depressed people used the two positive styles far less than the non-depressed people. One interesting fact that came out of this study is that there was no distinct correlation between either group and the aggressive humor style, meaning that depressed people are not genetically prone to this style any more than nondepressed people. What it also tells me is that people who use this style of humor do so by conscious choice. Now this study raises the question whether the proclivity to use self-defeating humor is a byproduct of the depression diagnosis or genetically underpinned, but one thing is exceedingly clear—humor is not a viable coping mechanism, unless it is of the "light" variety. The use of self-defeating humor as a stress reducer can have exceedingly negative effects and should be avoided. It's not known if the chicken or the egg crossed the road first, meaning are depressed people drawn to darker humor because of their depression or is there a genetic element at play behind the curtain? Who cares. In my world, it doesn't matter. If it adds to our darkness or costs us any of our valuable self-respect, then it has to go, period.

The big question that there is no concrete, scientific answer for is, can I change my style of humor? Let's take a step back and look at the bigger picture for just a minute. Above all else, I want you to be who you are, I want you to stand up tall and shout your truth, and I want you to be authentic and happy, to live long and prosper. I cannot tell you that and at the same time tell you to change, because that would make me a confusing dick. I would say that if you are using self-defeating humor to cope with stress, please consider finding another way; you are far too important to be continually minimizing yourself and you need to get to a place where you see that. Never willingly diminish your self-worth in order to put a smile on anyone else's face. If it gives you a feeling of accomplishment and purpose to put a smile on someone's face, then by all means follow that path but don't do it at the cost of your own dignity or self-respect.

Something to be aware of is that many depressed people may not feel that they have a sense of humor at all, that they only have a sense of seriousness, and it's overdeveloped. In my totally unprofessional and highly humorless opinion, there can be a reason for that. If that study is correct, the two "light" styles of humor may not resonate with you, and you may simply not be comfortable with the use of self-defeating humor, which would leave you solidly without humor style options, not without the capacity for humor. If you choose to redefine your style of humor, keep in mind that it's merely a form of communication, and like any other form, with hard work and a mindful approach, it can be manipulated and learned. Even though there may be some genetics involved, and a tendency to lean toward the dark side of humor, behavior can be changed or modified.

There is no tried or true recipe for creating or enhancing your sense of humor, no pill that will make others around you spontaneously laugh, but there are some things that you can work on that may bear dividends as time goes on. First things first, there is a difference between being funny and a sense of humor. Being funny means that you have the ability to express humor, nothing more. You can copy someone who is funny and make people laugh, but that doesn't give you a sense of humor, which is personal and developed by your experiences and unique world view.

That being said, your personal style will revolve around what makes you laugh, and for a lot of people who suffer from depression, they may have no idea whatsoever of what that is. Connecting with humor is vital to the process, so take as long as you need, watch something funny on Netflix if you can find anything, or Google "funny" and see what adventure awaits, but take a dive into the deep end of the humor pool and see if anything grabs you in your giggly place.

Once you learn to laugh, there are three broad categories that will help you incorporate humor more into your life. The first thing you have already begun and that is to bring more funny and comical things into your life. Make laughing a daily occurrence. No matter the darkness around you, find something to laugh at even if it doesn't feel natural at first and you feel you have to force it a little. It will be worth it if for nothing else to say a hearty "fuck you" to your depression. The next category is to start seeing humor in the world around you. Believe me, once you stop crying, you see the grand comedy that we are all playing a role in. Once you have completed these two things, you "officially" have a sense of humor or at the very least a better, more comical outlook than you previously held.

That, however, is not the end of the funny story. The third category is not actually required and is the most difficult of the three, which is learning how to translate your sense of humor to other people. This is where a sense of humor gives way to being funny. This category, however, comes with risk and consequence, so care should be taken in the implementation. Believe me, I've spent nights writhing in the agony of self-inflicted shit-in-mouth disease, with permanent facepalm disorder. You have to practice. Start small and always know your audience.

I want you to feel just as confident in displaying your sense of humor as in telling your story, but with either, it takes time, perseverance, and a lot of goddamn effort. Start with a close friend or somebody who you are comfortable with, then build upon successes and learn from failures. Know that with humor and its individualistic nature that there will come a time when upon telling a joke or what you feel is a humorous anecdote all that will be audible is the sounds of crickets and awkwardness. It will happen, and you will overcome it. Don't let that stop you; don't ever stop. A sense of humor, a positive "light" self-supporting sense of humor, is vital to your life and your fight and is more important than you may ever fully appreciate.

I think you would agree that Mahatma Gandhi had been through some shit. He was a lawyer, an anticolonial nationalist, a

Epilogue

Hello, it's so good to talk to you again. I know for you it's been like three seconds, but for me it's been weeks and weeks. I wanted to take a minute and tell you about how it's been going since we've been apart. Bill passed away, and as hard as it was to say goodbye, his passing was peaceful, his fight is over and he is enjoying the rest that he so deserves. Nancy is doing as good as can be expected given the situation. I still have depression, big surprise, but I have been working through it, continuing the meditation and contemplation that have changed my life. I have experienced PTSD since we last spoke, but the severity and duration has been diminished to a degree. I still haven't dealt with Josh's guilt or my Mom's unfulfilled promise, but feel like I'm getting stronger every day. In saying that the last thing I will share with you is the suicide note that I was going to leave for Lisa, I will never, ever, need it. I love you.

Lisa,

If your reading this it's because I'm gone and I know that nothing that I say will matter right now, maybe not for a long time, or ever, but I need to tell you some things and hope that someday they will matter and help make sense of the senseless.

I know this doesn't help but I'm sorry. I'm sorry for leaving you and the boys. I feel like I've brought nothing to our relationship but pain and suffering. You need someone who will take care of you how you deserve to be taken care of and the boys need someone who will be there who won't drag them down with his own problems. I'm tired in my soul, I'm tired of the pain that I feel, tired of seeing and feeling darkness all around me like I'm cursed. I tried to be that strong person for you but like a lot of things in my life, I failed.

There is so much that I want to tell you before I go but it's so hard. I can't say goodbye, I can't do it with my mouth, and so I'll write it down like a coward and hope that I can get through it.

To you, the love of my life, and I truly mean that, I have never loved another person like I have loved you. Since the moment I saw you in your Lane sweatpants I've wanted to be close to you and I thank God for the ability to share my life with you. I wanted so much to grow old with you, I'm just not strong enough.

Mack, I have to go, I'm sorry. You're a good boy and I know that you will grow up to be a good man. I want you to know that giving up is never good and I really wanted to stay with you but I couldn't. I'm sure you will grow to be a much stronger man than I was. Please take care of your mom, do what she tells you to do and protect your brothers. Know that I always love you and you've done nothing wrong, don't ever think that you did.

Joshua, I don't know how much of this you will understand. I want you to know that I'm sorry for everything I've done wrong for you, I really wish that I could have done more. I hope in some way that you realize how much I love you and how proud I have always been of you, I'm sorry.

Noah, my sweet little man. I'm sorry that I won't be there to watch you grow up. I know that you will have challenges but I know that you will find your strength in who you are. The thought of not seeing you and your brothers hurts me but I know you'll be in a better place than I could give you.

To my parents, to my sister Julie, to my brother Gary, I want you all to know that this is not your fault. I know you will feel guilty but this is only my decision. I love you all and thank you for being the best family that a person could ever have.

I know that nobody will understand this, I've tried hard to be tough to make it work but it's too much for me, too much pain. I'm drowning.

I'm sorry.

Rodger Deevers

About the Author

Rodger Deevers works in a family-owned financial services business and has been a lifelong depression sufferer. Rodger recently went into a PTSD induced break from reality and emerged with a story and a desire to change the negative stigma-driven narrative by which the world views depression and mental illness. It is Rodger's fondest wish that in some small way, *You, Therapy* will initiate a dialogue that offers insight to those who do not suffer and hope for those who do.